Understanding Self-Harm and Suicide for Nurses and Health Practitioners

This practical book equips nurses and health practitioners with essential knowledge and skills for understanding and supporting people experiencing suicidal thoughts and engaging in self-harm.

Exploring why people might experience suicidal ideation or feelings, or use self-harm, this skills-based book emphasises core skills a health practitioner needs to respond effectively and compassionately, dispelling myths and misconceptions that fuel stigma. It is informed throughout from service user perspectives and includes examples of good practice, suggestions for small changes that make meaningful differences, and reflective activities.

Promoting practice that enables people experiencing suicidal thoughts and engaging in self-harm to feel safer and more hopeful and to function at their best, this guide is an essential read for all health professionals.

Sarah Housden qualified as an occupational therapist in 1993 and has held positions promoting mental and physical health across charitable, private, and NHS settings with adults of all ages. Since 2014, she has worked at the University of East Anglia as an Associate Professor in Health Sciences where she aims to provide effective learning opportunities for pre- and post-qualifying nurses and allied health professionals through stimulating empathy and compassion for service users and patients. Additionally, she works part-time in the community for a charitable organisation to maintain awareness of issues affecting people every day in modern society and contemporary healthcare practice.

Essential Mental Health Skills for Nurses and Allied Health Professionals
Series Editor: Sarah Housden

Trauma-Informed Care for Nurses and Allied Health Professionals
Sarah Housden

Understanding Self-Harm and Suicide for Nurses and Health Practitioners
Sarah Housden

Understanding Self-Harm and Suicide for Nurses and Health Practitioners

Edited By
Sarah Housden

R Routledge
Taylor & Francis Group

LONDON AND NEW YORK

Designed cover image: Getty Images

First published 2026
by Routledge
4 Park Square, Milton Park, Abingdon, Oxon OX14 4RN

and by Routledge
605 Third Avenue, New York, NY 10158

Routledge is an imprint of the Taylor & Francis Group, an informa business

British Library Cataloguing-in-Publication Data
A catalogue record for this book is available from the British Library

Library of Congress Cataloging-in-Publication Data
Names: Housden, Sarah editor
Title: Understanding self-harm and suicide for nurses and health practitioners / edited by Sarah Housden.
Description: Abingdon, Oxon; New York, NY: Routledge, 2026. |
Series: Essential mental health skills for nurses and allied health professionals |
Includes bibliographical references and index. |
Identifiers: LCCN 2025044345 | ISBN 9781041064824 hardback |
ISBN 9781041064817 paperback | ISBN 9781003635611 ebook
Subjects: LCSH: Suicide | Suicidal behavior | Parasuicide
Classification: LCC RA1136 .U53 2026 | DDC 362.28—dc23/eng/20260206
LC record available at https://lccn.loc.gov/2025044345

ISBN: 978-1-041-06482-4 (hbk)
ISBN: 978-1-041-06481-7 (pbk)
ISBN: 978-1-003-63561-1 (ebk)

DOI: 10.4324/9781003635611

Typeset in Optima
by codeMantra

Contents

Contents

List of Tables, Figures and Boxes

Tables

Figures

Boxes

About the Contributors

Hannah Bailey qualified as a Mental Health Nurse in 2014, graduating from the University of East Anglia. Following her qualification, she went straight into working in Community Mental Health Care as a lead care professional/care coordinator, working with a broad range of complex clients. In 2020, she trained as a DBT Therapist with British Isles DBT and, following this, topped up her intensive training with Bangor University, completing a Post-Graduate Diploma. Since 2020, Hannah has supported the implementation and rollout of the Complex Emotional Needs Pathway in Norwich and worked as a DBT Therapist within Community Mental Health.

Louise Cherrill qualified as a mental health nurse at the University of East Anglia in 2018 and has worked in adult community, youth community, and community triage, access, and assessment teams in the NHS. She has completed intensive training in Dialectical Behavioural Therapy (PgCert) with British Isles DBT and Bangor University, and an MSc in Clinical Research. She is a clinical academic, working for the University of East Anglia (UEA) teaching pre-registration nursing as a mental health nursing lecturer, and in the NHS as a Senior Community Mental Health Practitioner. Louise is passionate about management of self-harm and suicidal behaviours, with this being the focus of her PhD. She has a particular interest in working to improve the experiences of service users accessing care, and in prevention of self-harm by mitigating risks as a public health agenda.

Sarah Housden qualified as an occupational therapist in 1993 and has held positions promoting mental and physical health across charitable, private, and NHS settings with adults of all ages. Since 2014, she has worked at the University of East Anglia as an Associate Professor in Health Sciences where she aims to provide effective learning opportunities for pre- and post-qualifying nurses and allied health professionals through stimulating their empathy and compassion for service users and patients. Additionally, she works part-time in the community for a charitable organisation to ensure she maintains awareness of issues affecting everyday people in modern society and contemporary healthcare practice.

John Whitebrook lost his youngest son, aged 26, to suicide in 2017. As a PhD biologist, he spent 30+ years in the pharmaceutical industry, primarily in drug safety. After retiring from the pharmaceutical industry, he has returned to studying, completing a Psychology Conversion MSc and embarking on a PhD in psychology at the University of West London. His current research is focused on postvention uptake and effectiveness in UK & Ireland adult male suicide loss survivors. He has had papers on postvention, including one describing a Suicide Bereavement Model, published in peer-reviewed journals, and co-authored the suicide bereavement support section of a British Standard: BS 30480 Suicide and the Workplace – Intervention, Prevention, and Support for People Affected by Suicide – Guide. John is a member of the International Association for Suicide Prevention Postvention Special Interest Group.

As well as being an active volunteer, co-facilitating peer support group meetings, he is Vice Chair of the Board of Trustees at Survivors of Bereavement by Suicide (SoBS), a charity dedicated to supporting suicide loss survivors. His remit includes driving and coordinating the charity's research involvement.

Series Preface

Essential Mental Health Skills for Nurses and Allied Health Professionals offers a series of books on key topics aimed at equipping non-specialist mental health practitioners with knowledge, skills, and understanding about the causes of mental and emotional distress, alongside tools for responding to people in their care who may be distressed or at risk of coming to harm due to a deterioration in their mental health.

Mental health presentations are increasingly evident across all areas of health and care provision, while specialist mental health services sometimes find it difficult to manage and respond to growing expressions of need amongst the population. This has resulted in an exponential growth in the demands made on general health and care practitioners to respond to people in mental and emotional distress, often in the absence of the timely availability of specialist mental health services with the capacity to respond swiftly.

Within this series, readers will be able to explore the interplay between a variety of factors contributing to mental ill-health, as they reflect on case studies of people with lived experience. These case studies are provided alongside more theoretical content and practical tools for immediate use, as well as information on more specialist therapeutic approaches and longer-term strategies for improving services. Theoretical ideas with examples of application to practice, followed by questions for reflection and discussion, provide practitioners, students, and educators with opportunities to consider their own values and beliefs in the light of research, theory, and evidence-based practice.

While acknowledging the challenges of contemporary healthcare practice, the series aims to support health and care practitioners to better understand the viewpoints of service users and thus to move towards developing a more empathic and compassionate approach to working with people living with mental health-related illnesses and other signs of stress and distress.

The books in this series are written for nurses and allied health professionals who are seeking an enhanced understanding of mental health to support their ongoing professional development as well as their clinical practice with patients and service users who are experiencing distress. It has been one of the highlights of my career as an academic, which I hope to enhance through this book series, to see health practitioners of all professions come to new understandings of people experiencing mental distress, leading to more empathic and compassionate approaches to healthcare delivery.

It is equally important to note that the world of healthcare is not neatly divided into people who have mental health problems and those who are here to support them. There is no "us" and "them" in healthcare: health practitioners are just as likely to have experienced trauma and to be living with mental distress, as those with whom they work. This is reflected in the fact that many of us who have authored chapters within this series are people who have a mixture of expertise by experience (as carers and service users) alongside being people who have acquired expertise through study and by working as healthcare practitioners, researchers, and academics. It is also worth noting that some of the case studies in this series are written by the editing and authorship team, based on our anonymised personal experiences as service users. This moves us beyond a tokenistic inclusion of the voices of service users to the meaningful production of a series of books which integrate service user expertise, just as it is integrated into our everyday lives and workplaces.

Dr Sarah Housden
Series Editor
June 2025

Introduction

Sarah Housden

As part of the "Essential Mental Health Skills for Nurses and Allied Health Professionals" series, this book's focus on self-harm and suicide provides a wealth of greatly needed tools and information for use in everyday health and social care practice, with the aim of equipping and empowering both you as the reader and the patients and service users with whom you work.

At the point of somebody presenting with, or disclosing self-harm to us, we may have a range of thoughts and feelings. We may question why they have done this, how they expect us to react, and how evidence-based practice or our code of professional conduct, say that we should react as healthcare practitioners. Personal thoughts and feelings may conflict with professional expectations, even more so when the person in question is a friend, family member or colleague.

In a busy healthcare system, it seems understandable on one level that healthcare practitioners may experience some feelings of resentment when treating a person who has self-harmed, when there are so many other people who are perceived as "more deserving" waiting for treatment.

One of our hopes in writing this book is that we can better equip health and care practitioners to understand, and be compassionate towards, people who have sometimes struggled for decades with emotional turmoil arising from adverse events and trauma that have occurred earlier in life. While self-harm is not the best coping mechanism, it may well be the only strategy the individual has available, through no fault of their own. In some situations, self-harm may be the least damaging of a range of options that the person thinks of carrying out, most of which are aimed at managing unbearable feelings and carrying on with life.

DOI: 10.4324/9781003635611-1

Our habitual ways of thinking about people who self-harm can be confirmed through unconscious bias or may be challenged when we put aside judgement and consider the needs of the person in front of us. For some people reading this book, self-injurious actions may be something they have thought about or engaged with on a personal level. It is essential to understand that this is not a situation where there are clear delineations between non-self-harming healthcare practitioners who are called upon to work with self-harming lay people. Depending on your experience and life history, you, or your colleagues, could be people who have historically used, or currently use, self-harm as a way of coping when work or your personal life does not seem to be manageable in any other way. The degree of stigma around self-harm means that many people will keep these actions hidden. The chances of this may be even greater when an individual works in a profession or setting where they witness people who self-harm being judged or blamed for their situations.

Some healthcare practitioners will express frustration that they need to spend time in their already-busy clinics, supporting people who, it would seem, have intentionally harmed themselves. Historically, the use of the term "deliberate self-harm" held intonations of blame, sometimes with anger and frustration, perhaps even disgust, more or less openly expressed towards people presenting to health services in need of support in managing their resulting injuries.

Changes in the language used to describe self-harm are an important part of improving services for people who injure themselves with or without suicidal intent. Evolving best practice has involved a move away from the sometimes accusatory-sounding term "deliberate self-harm" and the use of phrases like "superficial self-harm", which are recognised as unhelpful and as being used in ways that suggest that the person's distress and actions do not need to be taken seriously.

More important than the language used are changes in attitudes and understanding. Recognising the part played by emotional and psychological trauma, some of which may have occurred as part of adverse childhood events (Housden, 2025), is essential for recognising the origin of some self-injurious actions. Likewise, recognising that the majority of people injuring themselves, far from being attention seeking, are actually trying to manage feelings and experiences that are completely intolerable (NHS England Digital, 2025), with some saying that they have self-harmed as a way of reducing suicidal ideation and intent.

Similarly, the language used around suicide may not be ideal, where the term "committed suicide" is linked with a time in the past when suicidal actions were a crime. Suicide was decriminalised under the 1961 Suicide Act, but the criminal implication is still evident in the language sometimes used today in contemporary practice (NSPCC Learning, 2024). Likewise, terms like "successful suicide" suggest achievement. Instead, we need to focus on using objective but compassionate language such as "died by suicide". For those with suicidal thoughts, rather than saying that they are "suicidal", which can potentially define and limit our understanding of the whole person, it is more helpful to say that they are "experiencing thoughts of suicide".

In putting together the chapters of this book, we are keen that nurses, allied health professionals, and others involved in supporting people at times of distress, who do not have expertise gained through specialist mental health training, will be able to gain new information, understanding of theories and of approaches to working with patients and service users, alongside tools for practice, which will make a real difference to you and those with whom you work.

Chapter 1 provides an initial overview of self-harm and suicide, aimed at stimulating thinking and reflection about some of the factors that may not be obvious, or about which you may have wondered when working with individual patients and service users. In Chapter 2, Louise Cherrill begins to explore in more detail the idea of emotional regulation and some of the ways we can support people where emotions become dysregulated and difficult to manage. Louise then explores Stress and Distress in Chapter 3, presenting and reflecting on a range of ideas, including the need for risk assessment where expressed emotions are a cause for concern. Chapter 4 brings non-suicidal self-harm to the fore, as Louise Cherrill and Hannah Bailey explore key issues related to the causes and management of self-harm.

The final three chapters of the book focus more closely on suicide. In Chapter 5, Hannah Bailey looks into suicidal thoughts and how best to support people to manage these. This is followed by further work from Hannah, joined again by Louise in Chapter 6, as they consider how to help people find reasons to go on living, during an emotional or mental health crisis. Finally, in Chapter 7, John Whitebrook provides an exploration and presentation of the experiences of people who are bereaved when someone close to them dies by suicide. Included in John's chapter are some pertinent thoughts about how healthcare practitioners are affected when someone they have supported dies by suicide, alongside a sensitively presented explanation of the needs of bereaved families and friends.

As you read each of these chapters, you will notice that the terminology used to describe those who live with mental and emotional distress includes terms such as service user and patient. Although for practical purposes, a decision was made to adopt these specific descriptive terms, we would not want anyone to feel defined by these descriptions and believe that all people have the right to describe their relationship to service providers and to their own experiences, in whatever way feels most comfortable and appropriate to them. As authors, we also believe that there is no "them" and "us" in healthcare, as we all have the potential to become patients and service users at some point in our lives.

It is hoped that this book, along with other volumes in the 'Essential Mental Health Skills for Nurses and Allied Health Professionals' series, will play a key role in the education and professional development of nurses and allied health professionals going forward. The development of knowledge, understanding, and skills for practice will be enhanced through readers' active engagement with the questions for reflection and discussion, together with the suggestions for further reading, which you will find towards the end of each chapter. These will, ideally, be used for personal as well as team reflection and follow-up learning.

The authors and editor have produced this book in the hope that it will make a difference to you in promoting confidence and advancing your competence in interacting with people who have experienced emotional distress and mental ill-health. Ultimately, our aim is that this will in turn lead to benefits for you, your service users and patients, for the teams you are part of, and for the organisations for which you work.

Note on the Case Studies

The case studies in each chapter have been anonymised, with all identifying features altered or removed.

A Note on Self-Care

Reading about other people's experiences of distress can potentially trigger emotions and memories for anyone – whether we are healthcare practitioners

Table I.1 Sources of Support in a Crisis *(Correct at the Time of Publication)*

UK helpline numbers		
Mind	0300 102 1234	9 am–6 pm Monday – Friday
Samaritans	116 123	24 hours a day 365 days a year
SANEline	0300 304 7000	4:30 pm–10:00 pm daily
National Suicide Prevention Helpline	0800 689 5652	6 pm–midnight daily
SHOUT	Text SHOUT to: 85258	24/7 text service
NHS	111 Option 2	24 hours a day 365 days a year

or not. Please be mindful of this and take good care of yourself. In Chapter 6, we provide a table of Helpline Numbers, which may be equally helpful to healthcare professionals, patients, and service users. Useful contact numbers are given below for ease of access and are repeated in Chapter 6. Do not hesitate to speak to someone and reach out for help if you need to.

References

Housden, S. (2025). *Trauma-informed Practice for Nurses and Allied Health Professionals*. Abingdon: Routledge.

NHS England Digital (2025). Chapter 4: Suicidal thoughts, suicide attempts and non-suicidal self-harm - adult psychiatric morbidity survey: Survey of mental health and wellbeing, England. 2023/4. Available online at: https://digital.nhs.uk/data-and-information/publications/statistical/adult-psychiatric-morbidity-survey/survey-of-mental-health-and-wellbeing-england-2023-24/suicidal-thoughts-suicide-attempts-and-self-harm. [Accessed 18th August 2025].

NSPCC Learning (2024). 'Why language matters: Rethinking the language of suicide'. Available online at: https://learning.nspcc.org.uk/news/why-language-matters/rethinking-language-suicide. [Accessed 18th August 2025].

Suicide Act (1961). Available online at: https://www.legislation.gov.uk/ukpga/Eliz2/9-10/60. [Accessed 18th August 2025].

Self-Harm and Suicide

An Overview

Sarah Housden

Case Study

Katherine's Story

I remember the day my self-harming began, just as well as I remember the day it ended.

I was in my third year at secondary school and was experiencing some difficult things in my home and family life, which I felt completely unable to discuss with anyone. I had tried speaking to a couple of close friends at one point about my dad having attempted suicide. He was an in-patient in the local psychiatric hospital at the time. I really needed my friends to understand what I was going through; I needed some care and support. So, I said about him being unwell and in hospital. They were all ears and sympathy until I said the name of the hospital, and then they broke down in fits of giggles, pointing at me and saying: "Your dad's a looney!" They then ran off and I could hear them chanting as they ran: "Kath's dad's a looney! Kath's dad's a looney!" So much for getting any support from my closest friends.

It was a couple of weeks after that, and I was sitting on the school field at lunch time with a bunch of girls I didn't mix with so often. One of them, Sue, who was generally considered to be the ringleader, was showing the other girls how to cut themselves with their own fingernail. I watched, fascinated, having no idea why anyone would want to do this. Then Sue turned to me, saying: "What about you Kath – are you going to have a go? Or are you too scared?" Having avoided my closest friends since telling them about Dad being unwell, I was keen to be part

---

DOI: 10.4324/9781003635611-2

of another group of friends, and Sue' s encouragement to hurt myself, whilst perplexing, seemed like an obvious way into this new group.

So, I did it, and the amazing thing was, that as I began to pierce the skin on my hand, it felt like all my intense worries about my family, just melted away. So, this was what I was looking for – I didn't need to make new friends or hold onto the old ones even. Who cared whether anyone understood? I felt myself relax on the inside and knew that I had found a way of managing the intensity of emotions which had been consuming me with all their dark and destructive potential.

And as I said, I remember the day I stopped self-harming too. It was 20 years later. I was living in a bedsit, alone and with very few, if any, friends. I was 35 and had not worked for the past ten years. The only things of note in my diary were appointments with health professionals who, after ten years of input, were no closer to being able to reduce the strength of my suicidal thoughts and intentions. So, I lurched from crisis to crisis, in-patient stay to in-patient stay, managing my almost compulsive thoughts about suicide and preventing myself from acting on these, by continuing to harm myself. Over the years, the cutting had become much more secretive. From that first cut on the hand which everyone seemed to notice and ask about, much to my embarrassment, I learned to cut in more discreet places which remained hidden by clothing. It was my secret tool, that I used to keep myself alive, regardless of everything inside me that was telling me to end my life.

So, there I am, 20 years after that first cut, and I'm hanging over the bath, as usual, to prevent blood from staining the carpet. And suddenly, out of nowhere, I think to myself: "This isn't actually helping". And that one self-generated but wholly realistic thought, was the beginning of the end as far as cutting was concerned, for me.

It's now over 30 years later, and I've recently retired from paid work. Looking back, I am so grateful to that part of myself that spoke to my inner self that day. It was helpful that the questioning came from me, rather than yet another person advising me against it. I found it within myself to query the effectiveness of the ongoing use of self-harm as a way of managing my emotional turmoil, even though it had prevented suicidal thoughts turning into actions on numerous occasions. I can't say that I've never thought about harming myself it since then, but I've never wanted to do it like I did before, and I no longer see it as a sustainable way of coping with my darkest feelings, even though they still plague me from time to time.

Introduction

Suicidal thoughts and actions, as well as non-suicidal self-injury, are associated with significant distress for the people who experience them, as well as for their families, friends, and the healthcare practitioners who support them. Although there is an association with diagnosed mental health conditions, self-harm and suicide can also be experienced by people without any diagnosed condition (NHS England Digital, 2025).

In 2023, the suicide rate reached its highest figure since 1999, with 6,069 suicides registered in England and Wales. That is 11.4 deaths per 100,000 people (Office for National Statistics, 2024), with each life lost affecting many more people in their surrounding network of family, friends, healthcare professionals, and work colleagues, in profound and lasting ways.

Chapter Aims

This chapter provides an overview of key issues around self-harm and suicide, including information and ideas which explore:

- What we mean by self-harm and suicide, and who is likely to be affected.
- Considerations around social and cultural differences in understandings of self-harm and suicide.
- The hidden figures and some of the barriers to seeking and gaining relevant support and care.
- Approaches that healthcare practitioners can adopt to better support people in the short term.
- Society- and system-level changes which could potentially address the needs of people who self-harm and so contribute to a reduction in the number of people who die by suicide.

What Is Self-Harm and Why Does It Take Place?

When we talk about self-harm or non-suicidal self-injury, we are talking about actions which individuals carry out, for purposes which may or may not be known to them and those around them. Self-harming actions such as cutting, burning, or hitting oneself used to be viewed as self-mutilation and a form of "attenuated suicide" (Hooley et al., 2020). The term non-suicidal self-injury differentiates clearly between self-inflicted harm that is intended to be fatal and self-inflicted harm that is used as a coping strategy – effectively being a strategy to survive, not to die (Rayner and Wright, 2023).

NICE (2025) defines self-harm as "an intentional act of self-poisoning or self-injury, irrespective of the motivation or apparent purpose of the act and is an expression of emotional distress". Self-injurious actions are an expression of personal distress, and it is important to note that they are also a risk factor for a person subsequently ending their life through suicide (Duarte et al., 2020). Following an episode of self-harm, suicide risk is significantly increased, particularly in people who have repeatedly self-harmed, are male, have expressed suicidal intentions, and have physical health problems (NICE, 2025).

How Prevalent Is Self-Harm?

Population-level surveys provide the most accurate measure of the national prevalence of self-harm, as they capture data directly from the public, regardless of whether an individual has sought medical care. These data establish a baseline for understanding the scale of the issue that is not necessarily reflected in official statistics derived from data collected across statutory services.

The findings from population-level surveys suggest that, within the UK, the prevalence of self-harm has risen significantly over the past two decades. The proportion of 16- to 74-year-olds reporting lifetime self-harm has increased from 2.4% in 2000 to 6.4% in 2014, and further still, to 10.3% in 2023/2024 (NHS England Digital, 2025). This upward trend is not unique to self-harm but reflects a consistent rise across a broad range of common mental health conditions, which increased from 18.9% in 2014 to 22.6% in 2023/2024. At the same time, the proportion of 16- to 74-year-olds reporting suicidal thoughts in the past year has also risen from 3.8% in 2000 to 6.7% in 2023/2024, with past-year suicide attempts rising from 0.5 to 1.0% over the same period (NHS England Digital, 2025). Taken together, these data indicate a growing issue, for which healthcare practitioners need to be trained and equipped to respond confidently, competently, and with compassion.

However, the available data are somewhat fragmented, and it is challenging to attempt to gain a comprehensive understanding of the extent of, and specific patterns within, incidents of self-harm in the United Kingdom. Official statistics from primary, secondary, and emergency services provide a valuable but incomplete picture, capturing only those individuals who present to health services for care and support. There is also a significant number of "hidden" people needing consideration, who do not seek help, and who keep their self-harm and suicidal ideation largely to themselves (Knipe et al., 2022). While the prevalence of self-injurious actions in the general population is rising, official service-level data for hospital admissions are decreasing. There is, therefore, a recognised gap between the need for, and access to, expert care.

Emergency Services and Hospital Admissions

While population surveys capture the overall scale of self-harm, an analysis of service presentation data provides a measure of the demands this is placing on the UK's healthcare system. Emergency departments and hospital admissions for self-harm are a key measure of acute mental health crises happening in our communities. It is estimated that there are 220,000 emergency department presentations and around 110,000 hospital admissions annually in England, as a result of self-harm (Department of Health and Social Care, 2024).

Analysing the data by age group reveals some patterns. A 2019 systematic review and meta-analysis of global data between 1989 and 2018 showed that the proportion of children and adolescents who had ever engaged in non-suicidal self-injury was 22.1%, while the 12-month prevalence was 19.5% (Lim et al., 2019). This meta-analysis found that non-suicidal self-injury, suicidal ideation, and deliberate self-harm were the three most common suicidal and self-harm behaviours in children and adolescents. A 2022 systematic review and meta-analysis of data dealing with suicide or self-harm in children aged under 12 years reported that the pooled prevalence from four studies was 1.4% and was similar for both sexes (Geoffroy et al., 2022).

There is a suggestion of a shifting burden of self-harm towards younger cohorts, although we must also maintain awareness that self-harm is a potential issue regardless of age group. Sachs-Ericsson et al. (2016) found an association between suicidal thoughts and intentions in later life and adverse childhood events which had taken place several decades earlier.

Primary Care Presentations

For many individuals, the general practitioner is the first point of contact for help with self-harm, making primary care a vital frontline service (Mughal et al., 2020). Research indicates that presentations to general practice of people who have self-harmed are increasing. For example, a large-scale study of primary care data from 2001 to 2013 found increasing presentation rates over time for both genders, even as the incidence trend for females remained stable. This study also revealed a decreasing gradient of risk with increasing age and a markedly elevated risk for females aged 15–24, who had presentation rates 3.75 times higher than all other females (Cybulski et al., 2022).

Another finding from primary care research is the significant gap between the number of people seeking help and those being referred to a specialist. Despite the high burden on services, one study found that only 15.2% of patients with a self-harm episode were referred to mental health services (Carr et al., 2016), a referral gap that is compounded by health inequalities. Carr et al. (2016) also found that patients registered at practices in the most deprived localities were found to be 27.1% less likely to be referred than those in the least deprived areas. This finding is particularly concerning, given an established link between socioeconomic deprivation and self-harm (NICE, 2025). It indicates a systemic failure where the population with the greatest need is receiving the least specialised care, which could directly contribute to the escalating scale of unmet need. There is a potential suggestion in these data, that self-harming behaviours are less likely to be identified as problematic or unexpected, among people living in situations of socioeconomic advantage, such that, if a person from a family identified as being of a higher social class seeks support after an episode of self-harm, they are more likely to receive services from a specialist, thus increasing their chances of gaining more adaptive coping strategies at an early stage. Over time, an approach that makes a more socially and economically advantaged person more likely to get support is likely to accentuate the erroneous normalisation of self-harm among people from disadvantaged homes and families.

Hidden Figures: Barriers and Unmet Need

UK data suggest 60% of adults and 90% of young people aged 12–17 do not contact medical or psychological services after self-harming (Knipe et al., 2022). Alternative estimations suggest only 1 in 28 young men and 1 in 18 young women will seek professional help in these circumstances (Fenton and Kingsley, 2023).

A fundamental conclusion drawn from comparing population-level prevalence with service presentation data is the existence of a considerable, uncounted population of people who self-harm without seeking help from statutory services. Population surveys reveal that many of those who self-harm do not consult health services and, if they do, may not be perceived as needing ongoing support, or may not receive appropriate care. The disparity between a 10.3% lifetime prevalence rate (NHS England Digital, 2025) and the approximately 220,000 annual emergency department presentations highlights this profound unmet need (Department of Health and Social Care, 2024).

Some of the reasons behind this disparity include stigma, shame, fear, previous negative experiences when services have been approached for help, combined with systemic barriers (Mughal, 2022).

Stigma, Shame, and Secrecy

One deterrent to seeking help is the stigma and shame associated with self-harm. Keeping the self-harm and suicidal thoughts secret can lead to increased isolation and ongoing use of harmful coping mechanisms. Stigma can arise from public opinion, internalisation of negative thoughts about the self, as well as receiving some "not-so-kind" treatment from healthcare practitioners who have sometimes treated self-harming individuals as though they are "a waste of time". This kind of approach, sometimes taken towards individuals who are doing their very best to keep themselves alive in the context of suicidal thoughts, can be incredibly harmful to patients and service users, at a time when they already feel ashamed and vulnerable.

This can make it difficult to trust people and can act as a significant barrier to seeking help in the future.

Fear and Past Negative Experiences

Individuals may also experience fear of the potential consequences of disclosing self-harm. Young people, especially, may fear a loss of confidentiality or having their family informed without their consent. These fears can be rooted in past negative experiences with professionals, where expectations have not been met. Sometimes, health practitioners are perceived as relying too heavily on prescribed medication without exploring the root causes of distress. At other times, though, the opposite happens, and people experience their self-harm being casually dismissed as "minor" or "superficial" with a lack of care and understanding being offered at a time of immense distress. These sorts of experiences can make it difficult for people to try to get help again, thereby increasing the risk of lasting damage during future episodes of self-harm or suicidal thinking.

Systemic Barriers

Beyond personal and psychological factors, there are issues within the healthcare system that act as significant barriers to care. These include difficulties in accessing appropriate services in a timely manner. Long waiting times for mental health services are a common complaint from individuals seeking help, with many having to wait months for an initial appointment. This can lead to a deterioration in the person's condition and a compounding of their reliance on coping strategies that are harmful.

Socioeconomic and Financial Determinants

Evidence consistently demonstrates a strong link between self-harm and socioeconomic disadvantage. There is a clear gradient of increasing self-harm risk across deprivation quintiles, with a notable increase for those in the most deprived areas. Research indicates that the psychosocial factors contributing to self-harm are heavily clustered in the poorest localities (Samaritans, 2017), with national, local, and individual factors accumulating to trigger episodes of self-harm.

At a national level, the socioeconomic determinants most likely to increase the risk of suicidal behaviour in the population relate to times of economic recession and uncertainty, which are often times of high unemployment, coinciding with reduced levels of unemployment benefits and accompanied by sometimes harsh measures to deter benefit claimants. Within local communities, reduced opportunities for employment linked to the closure of local workplaces, alongside longstanding socioeconomic deprivation in that geographical area, add to a pervading sense of hopelessness which leads to increased risks of suicide (Samaritans, 2017). For individuals, socioeconomic determinants include unemployment, job insecurity, being in a manual occupation, along with having a low socioeconomic status due to poverty, poor educational attainment, and living in rented accommodation, especially in an area of deprivation (Samaritans, 2017).

So, it seems evident that the relationship between socioeconomic status and increased risk of suicide exists due to a compounding effect of multiple stressors. Research shows that economic hardships, such as unemployment, debt, and housing problems, can accumulate over time, before a triggering incident is experienced as the final straw and self-harm or suicide takes place. The greatest risks are presented where multiple stressors accumulate – such as debt and financial insecurity, on top of pre-existing mental health issues. This explains why periods of economic recession are often characterised by increases in self-harm and suicide, particularly among men who may perceive that they are experiencing a greater loss of social role, status, and income during times of economic downturn.

This compounding of factors highlights that for the reduction and prevention of self-harm and suicide, a holistic approach is necessary – one that addresses the underlying economic and social vulnerabilities that exist in modern society, as much as the social, psychological, and emotional needs of the individual.

Cultural and Social Considerations

Al-Sharifi et al. (2015) found that there are clear ethnic differences in self-harm and suicide, which may be affected by factors such as cultural pressures and prevalence of, or different understandings of, mental illness. Findings from this study included significant differences in the rates of self-harm between ethnic groups, with Asian males being least likely to self-harm and Black females being most likely. Factors that Al-Sharifi et al. found may help protect or predispose individuals to self-harm or suicide (such as religion, mental health, and coping styles) differed between ethnic groups. More recently, John (2022) found that unintentional injuries, sexual behaviours, adverse childhood experiences, health status, and poverty, alongside racial discrimination, were associated with self-harm and or suicidal ideation in ethnically diverse populations. Similarly, Freedland et al. (2024) found a three-way association between methods of self-harming, gender, and culture in a study that concluded that clinicians should consider culture and gender when assessing for suicide risk, because different intentions may be reflected in similar self-harming actions, depending on an individual's culture and gender.

The increasing availability of digital technology and social media has introduced new and complex issues around self-harm, particularly for young people. The internet represents both a useful source of supportive communities and resources for self-help, as well as being a platform overflowing with sometimes devastatingly harmful content, including pro-self-harm and pro-suicide material.

A recent study found that high levels of problematic mobile phone use and disturbed sleep were prevalent among young people with mental health conditions who self-harmed (Bye et al., 2024). While this research provides a strong association, it should be noted that a direct causal link has yet to be established. Nonetheless, the data highlight the need to understand the role of online environments in the lives of vulnerable young people.

There are also delicate social, cultural, and contextual factors that underpin the concept of self-harm, which determine when actions or patterns of behaviour are identified as self-harm and when they are not. For example, it has sometimes been said that tattoos are a form of self-harm as they permanently change an individual's appearance and can be a way of releasing and expressing emotions and feelings. However, tattoos are just as likely to be a means of positive self-expression, with many people appreciating body art, including tattoos and piercings, as a means of artistic expression, self-empowerment, and cultural significance, linked to an expression of beliefs, experiences, and identity. Therefore, while tattoos, piercings, and body modification represent the continuum of culturally and socially acceptable behaviours within the western society, they can also be understood in ways that meet the definitions of self-harm, in some instances.

Body Modification

Some forms of body modification are perceived as more extreme and socially unacceptable. A few examples of these will be explored here, together with explanations of what they involve. Play piercing involves inserting needles or other sharp objects into the skin, sometimes in patterns or designs, for a short period of time, and then removing them, allowing the wounds to heal. This can be done for aesthetic, ritualistic, or sexual reasons. Similarly, scarification has a long history in a range of cultures and is also practiced for aesthetic reasons in modern body modification. It involves marking the skin through cuts, burns, or branding – using designs, patterns, or images to permanently scar the body. This is a form of body art where the scars are deliberately created and manipulated to form raised or textured designs. Eyeball tattooing involves ink being injected into the white part of the eye to permanently change its colour. It is an especially controversial form of body art, due to its potential risks and irreversible nature. Lastly, suspension piercing is a form of body modification where large, sterilised hooks are pierced through the skin and then used to suspend a person in the air. It is a practice rooted in ancient rituals and is also a modern form of body modification that some people find cathartic, as well as a way of exploring their physical and mental limits.

These forms of body modification have been explored as a way of highlighting that while some types of self-harm are identified in a stigmatising way, as maladaptive coping strategies, other approaches which injure or change the appearance of the body, which may equally bring emotional release and catharsis, are identified as either fully or partially socially and culturally acceptable. It is also worth noting that some researchers (for example, Blay et al., 2023) have noted an association between body modification and non-suicidal self-injury amongst patients diagnosed with borderline personality disorder. In such instances, emotion regulation may be a link between both body modification and non-suicidal self-injury in the population studied.

Eating Disorders

In a somewhat more complex example, there are some forms of harming the self that are not necessarily considered through the same lenses, or with the same frameworks, as self-harm. An example of this is the harm to the self, caused by eating disorders. Research and practice guidelines about self-harm do not generally include eating disorders within the behaviours defined as self-harm, although Washburn et al. (2023) identified that behaviours associated with disordered eating, such as bingeing, purging, overexercising, or restricting food intake, may function as a form of non-suicidal self-injury. In their research, Washburn and colleagues found that among patients receiving partial hospitalisation or intensive outpatient treatment for non-suicidal self-injury, nearly one-third indicated engaging in disordered eating behaviours for the purpose of causing pain or damage to their bodies. They therefore recommend that healthcare services should consider assessing, and providing relevant interventions for, self-injurious disordered eating behaviours, alongside those behaviour patterns that are more traditionally identified as self-harming (Washburn et al., 2023).

Cucchi et al. (2016) identified that over one quarter of a sample of people living with eating disorders also engaged in non-suicidal self-injury. However, Kiekens and Claes (2020), while noting that NSSI and eating disorders frequently co-occur, also suggest that there is a need to further explore the longer-term developmental and the shorter-term momentary relationship of these behaviours in daily life. They identify an interaction between short- and long-term causes and triggers for both eating disorders and non-suicidal self-injury, highlighting that these are not actions that can be understood as being either impulsive or as a straightforward reaction to emotional stressors in the moment.

Normalised Harm?

Emotional regulation and the experience and expression of emotions are often portrayed in negative ways, but it is worth thinking about the stigmatising effects of identifying some forms of emotional regulation and expression as maladaptive, while normalising the actions of individuals (maybe ourselves or our colleagues) who come home from work feeling stressed and order a large pizza for our sole consumption, alongside drinking a bottle of wine, as a way of managing our stress. Indeed, the whole process of pathologising trauma by identifying self-harming behaviours as a symptom of a diagnosable mental health condition can be traumatising for some people, while for others, it can provide a welcome explanation of their personal experiences, which brings them comfort and a sense of understanding.

Tools for Now: Small Changes That Can Make a Big Difference

A key intervention which can help people to reduce or stop self-harming, and which can also turn a person away from suicidal actions, is a compassionate and understanding response from healthcare practitioners, as well as from family, friends, and other social contacts.

Seeing self-harm or the expression of suicidal thoughts as "attention-seeking" needs to be a thing of the past, which stays firmly in the past. If you find yourself thinking that an individual has injured themselves in order to gain attention from others, challenge yourself with the important questions of what needs this person has that are not being satisfactorily met, and what is leading them to this point of carrying out actions that we find challenging to treat and to support them with.

Encourage self-compassion among patients and service users by modelling and demonstrating compassion to them. Demonstrating empathy, understanding, and acceptance towards their experiences, while also encouraging them to cultivate these qualities within themselves, helps in reducing the self-criticism, shame, and isolation, which are often associated with self-harming behaviours (Rayner and Wright, 2023).

Equip individuals with self-soothing techniques, which may help them to reduce the intensity of feelings in the moment. While these techniques are not going to make underlying difficulties disappear, they can reduce the intensity of feelings in the moment and so avert compounding the crisis.

Lastly, be clear in your mind that not all people who self-harm do this forever. There are effective interventions, and our role is sometimes to equip and empower the individual to regulate their emotions and manage strong feelings until such time as they can access suitable longer-term interventions.

Self-Harm Reduction and Suicide Prevention: Systemic Approaches

There are several key findings that should inform the development of a strategy aimed at reducing the risk of harm caused by self-harm and suicide. These will be explored below.

The Prevalence–Presentation Gap

The national picture is one of a significant and continuing increase in self-harm, along with that of other common mental health conditions. Data suggesting a decrease in hospital admissions need to be interpreted cautiously, with recognition that it may be influenced by changes in reporting methods rather than reflecting an actual reduction in self-harming. A transparent reporting framework is needed to prevent misleading conclusions drawn from any changes in methodology, such as establishing a national, standardised data collection system to capture all presentations of self-harm. This needs to include emergency department attendances, rather than just hospital admissions, and to integrate these data with those collected in primary care settings.

Health Inequality and the Referral Gap

The lower referral rates for individuals from deprived areas, who are at a higher risk of self-harm, represent a clear case of health inequality. The healthcare system is not adequately reaching and supporting the most vulnerable populations, perpetuating a cycle of unmet need.

Substantial investment is required to reduce the unacceptably long waiting times for specialist mental health services. This should be coupled with a strategic shift of resources to areas of highest socioeconomic deprivation to address the referral gap and ensure equitable access to care.

Stigma and Fear

Stigma, shame, and fear of judgement – both from the public and, in some cases, from health and care practitioners – are frequently cited reasons why individuals do not seek help. This psychological barrier is as significant as any systemic or socioeconomic factor.

Campaigns to combat the pervasive stigma surrounding self-harm are worth considering. These would need to be informed by messages that focus on reframing self-harm as an expression of distress rather than a form of attention-seeking.

At the same time, all healthcare professionals, but particularly those in frontline roles in primary care and emergency departments, need evidence-based training on the assessment and compassionate management of people who have self-harmed. This training needs to address judgemental attitudes as well as provide skills for delivering trauma-informed care and understanding of potential referral routes for specialist support.

The Accumulation of Risk

Self-harm is not typically caused by a single trigger but occurs where there is a culmination of multiple, often compounding, factors. Socioeconomic hardships related to poverty, debt, and unemployment act as potent exacerbators of risk, particularly when combined with pre-existing mental health issues.

A comprehensive national strategy that integrates health policy with social and economic policy needs to be developed. Interventions should not be limited to clinical settings but must also address the root causes of self-harm, such as providing practical and therapeutic support for individuals experiencing unemployment and those living with overwhelming debt.

Addressing these systemic and social determinants of self-care and suicide is likely to move us towards a more accurate understanding of self-harm and suicide as a society. Only then can we begin to close the gap between public need and the availability of appropriate, compassionate, and life-changing care.

Summary of Learning Points

This chapter has provided some initial insights into what is meant by self-harm and suicide, providing a platform from which the following chapters will deliver a more in-depth exploration. In particular, it has provided an understanding of:

- Definitions of self-harm and suicide, including patterns among children and adolescents, as well as adults, with consideration being given to factors that may trigger self-harm for people of all ages.
- Social and cultural influences, including considerations of types of harm to self that are not traditionally included in research, policy, or guidelines relating to non-suicidal self-injury. Examples included a range of approaches to body modification, as well as exploring some of the complexities associated with harm to the self, caused by eating disorders.

- People whose self-harm or struggles with suicidal thoughts are hidden and the reasons behind this including shame, stigma, and fear.
- Compassionate and empathic approaches that healthcare practitioners can adopt to better support people presenting with self-harm or suicidal ideation.
- System-level changes that could potentially address the needs of people who self-harm and contribute to a reduction in the number of people who die by suicide, including improved data collection, training and increasing public awareness as a way of potentially reducing stigma.

Questions for Reflection and Discussion

1. Have you ever felt challenged by your feelings in the context of a patient or service user presenting to healthcare services after an episode of self-harm?

2. Following your reading of this chapter, are there any aspects of your own or any of your colleagues' thinking around self-harm and suicide that may need rethinking?

3. If approached for advice by a colleague or by a family member of a person who has self-harmed, what would you describe as being the best approach to take with the patient or service user?

4. Outline how non-suicidal self-injury differs from body modification practices, considering whether the way you speak to people presenting with skin infections due to either cause may need modifying.

5. Identify areas in which you need to increase your knowledge, understanding, and skills in relation to working with patients and service users affected by self-harm and suicide.

Recommended Follow-up Reading

Centre for Clinical Interventions (2019). Looking after yourself: Self compassion – workbook. Available online at: https://www.cci.health.wa.gov.au/resources/looking-after-yourself/self-compassion. [Accessed 20th August 2025].

Donnellan, C. (2000). *Self Harm and Suicide*. Cambridge, MA: Independence Educational Publishers.

Hibbins, J. (2021). *Suicide Prevention Guidebook: How to Support Someone Who Is Having Suicidal Feelings*. London: Trigger Publishing.

McEvoy, D., Brannigan, R., Cooke, L., Butler, E., Walsh, C., Arensman, E. and Clarke, M. (2023). Risk and protective factors for self-harm in adolescents and young adults: An umbrella review of systematic reviews. *Journal of Psychiatric Research*. 168: 353–380.

Richardson, R., Connell, T., Foster, M., Blamires, J., Keshoor, S., Moir, C. and Zeng, I.S. (2024). Risk and protective factors of self-harm and suicidality in adolescents: An umbrella review with meta-analysis. *Journal of Youth & Adolescence*. 53(6): 1301–1322.

References

Al-Sharifi, A., Krynicki, C.R. and Upthegrove, R. (2015). Self-harm and ethnicity: A systematic review. *International Journal of Social Psychiatry*. 61(6): 600–612.

Blay, M., Hasler, R., Nicastro, R., Pham, E., Weibel, S., Debbané, M. and Perroud, N. (2023). Body modifications in borderline personality disorder patients: Prevalence rates, link with non-suicidal self-injury, and related psychopathology. *Borderline Personality Disorder and Emotion Dysregulation*. 10(1): 1–11.

Bye, A., Carter, B., Leightley, D., Trevillion, K., Liakata, M., Branthonne-Foster, S., Cross, S., Zenasni, Z., Carr, E., Williamson, G., Viyuela, A.V. and Dutta, R. (2024). Cohort profile: The social media, smartphone use and self-harm in young people (3S-YP) study - a prospective, observational cohort study of young people in contact with mental health services. *PLoS ONE*. 19(5): e0299059.

Carr, M.J., Ashcroft, D.M., Kontopantelis, E., While, D., Awenat, Y., Cooper, J., Chew-Graham, C., Kapur, N. and Webb, R.T. (2016). Clinical management following self-harm in a UK-wide primary care cohort. *Journal of Affective Disorders*. 197: 182–188.

Cucchi, A., Ryan, D., Konstantakopoulos, G., Stroumpa, S., Kacar, A.S., Renshaw, S., Landau, S. and Kravariti, E. (2016). Lifetime prevalence of non-suicidal self-injury in patients with eating disorders: A systematic review and meta-analysis. *Psychological Medicine*. 46(7): 1345–1358.

Cybulski, L., Ashcroft, D.M., Carr, M.J., Garg, S., Chew-Graham, C.A., Kapur, N. and Webb, R.T. (2022). Risk factors for nonfatal self-harm and suicide among adolescents: two nested case-control studies conducted in the UK Clinical Practice Research Datalink. *Journal of Child Psychology and Psychiatry, and Allied Disciplines*. 63(9): 1078–1088.

Department and Health and Social Care (2024). Available online at: https://fingertips. phe.org.uk/search/self%20harm#page/4/gid/1/pat/159/par/K02000001/ati/ 15/are/E92000001/iid/21001/age/1/sex/4/cat/-1/ctp/-1/yrr/1/cid/4/tbm/1. [Accessed 18th August 2025].

Duarte, T.A., Paulino, S., Almeida, C., Gomes, H.S., Santos, N. and Gouveia-Pereira, M. (2020). Self-harm as a predisposition for suicide attempts: A study of adolescents' deliberate self-harm, suicidal ideation, and suicide attempts. *Psychiatry Research*. 287. 112553: 1–7.

Fenton, C. and Kingsley, E. (2023) Scoping review: Alternatives to self-harm recommended on mental health self-help websites. *International Journal of Mental Health Nursing*. 32(1): 76–94.

Freedland, A.S., Sundaram, K., Liu, N.H., Barakat, S., Muñoz, R.F. and Leykin, Y. (2024). Self-harm behaviors and their intentions: A cross-cultural analysis. *Journal of Mental Health*. 33(3): 295–303.

Geoffroy, M.C., Bouchard, S., Per, M., Khoury, B., Chartrand, E., Renaud, J., Turecki, G., Colman, I. and Orri, M. (2022). Prevalence of suicidal ideation and self-harm behaviours in children aged 12 years and younger: A systematic review and meta-analysis. *Lancet Psychiatry*. 9(9): 703–714.

Hooley, J.M., Fox, K.R. and Boccagno, C. (2020). Nonsuicidal self-injury: Diagnostic challenges and current perspectives. *Neuropsychiatric Disease and Treatment*. 16: 101–112.

John, L. (2022). Investigating the role of ethnicity and religion or spirituality on the risk of self-harm in children and adolescents: A systematic literature review. *BJPsych Open*. 8: S55–S56.

Kiekens, G. and Claes, L. (2020). Non-suicidal self-injury and eating disordered behaviors: An update on what we do and do not know. *Current Psychiatry Reports*. 22(12): 1–11.

Knipe, D., Padmanathan, P., Newton-Howes, G., Chan, L.F. and Kapur, N. (2022). Suicide and self-harm. *Lancet*. 399(10338): 1903–1916.

Lim, K.S., Wong, C.H., McIntyre, R.S., Wang, J., Zhang, Z., Tran, B.X., Tan, W., Ho, C.S. and Ho, R.C. (2019). Global lifetime and 12-month prevalence of suicidal behavior, deliberate self-harm and non-suicidal self-injury in children and adolescents between 1989 and 2018: A meta-analysis. *International Journal of Environmental Research and Public Health*. 16(22): 4581.

Mughal, F., Troya, M.I., Dikomitis, L., Chew-Graham, C.A., Corp, N. and Babatunde, O.O. (2020). Role of the GP in the management of patients with self-harm behaviour: A systematic review. *British Journal of General Practice*. 70(694): e364–e373.

Mughal, F., Dikomitis, L., Babatunde, O.O. and Chew-Graham, C.A. (2022). The potential of general practice to support young people who self-harm: A narrative review. *BJGP Open*. 6(1): 1–5.

NHS England Digital (2025). Chapter 4: Suicidal thoughts, suicide attempts and non-suicidal self-harm - adult psychiatric morbidity survey: Survey of mental health and wellbeing, England, 2023/4. Available online at: https://digital.nhs.uk/data-and-information/publications/statistical/adult-psychiatric-morbidity-survey/survey-of-mental-health-and-wellbeing-england-2023-24/suicidal-thoughts-suicide-attempts-and-self-harm. [Accessed 18th August 2025].

NICE (2025). Self-harm: What are the risk factors? Available online at: https://cks.nice.org.uk/topics/self-harm/background-information/risk-factors/. [Accessed 18th August 2025].

Office for National Statistics (2024). Suicides in England and Wales: 2023 registrations. Available online at: https://www.ons.gov.uk/peoplepopulationandcommunity/birthsdeathsandmarriages/deaths/bulletins/suicidesintheunitedkingdom/2023. [Accessed 18th August 2025].

Rayner, G. and Wright, K. (2023). Compassionate care for people who self-harm: Principles, tools and techniques. *Mental Health Practice*. 26(2): 34–41.

Sachs-Ericsson, N.J., Stanley, I.H., Sheffler, J. and Rushing, N.C. (2016). In my end is my beginning: Developmental trajectories of adverse childhood experiences to late-life suicide. *Aging and Mental Health*. 20(2): 139–165.

Samaritans (2017). Socioeconomic disadvantage and suicidal behaviour: Full Report Available online at: https://media.samaritans.org/documents/Socioeconomic_disadvantage_and_suicidal_behaviour_-_Full.pdf. [Accessed 18th August 2025].

Washburn, J.J., Soto, D., Osorio, C.A. and Slesinger, N.C. (2023). Eating disorder behaviors as a form of non-suicidal self-injury. *Psychiatry Research*. 319: 1–7.

2 | Approaches to Understanding and Regulating Emotions

Louise Cherrill

Case Study

Mika's Story

I've always had trouble managing my emotions. It's like I'm on a constant rollercoaster, which I can't seem to get off. For as long as I can remember, I've been overwhelmed by feelings of anger, sadness, and anxiety, often without any clear reason.

One of the most challenging experiences I've faced was during my final year of university. The pressure of assignments, exams, and the uncertainty of the future became too much for me. My emotions started to spiral out of control. I'd find myself crying uncontrollably or snapping at my friends and family over the smallest things. I felt like I was drowning in a sea of emotions, and I didn't know how to swim to the surface.

My inability to regulate my emotions affected my relationships. My friends started to distance themselves, unsure of how to help or react to my outbursts. My family, too, struggled to understand what I was going through. I felt isolated and alone, which only made things worse.

It wasn't until I sought help from a therapist that I began to understand the importance of emotional regulation. My therapist introduced me to Cognitive-Behavioural Therapy (CBT), which helped me identify and challenge my negative thought patterns. She also taught me mindfulness techniques to stay present and not get overwhelmed by my emotions.

One particularly helpful strategy was practising deep breathing exercises whenever I felt my emotions starting to spiral. I also started

DOI: 10.4324/9781003635611-3

journaling to express my feelings and gain clarity. Over time, I started noticing a difference. I still have my ups and downs, but I've learned to recognise the triggers and implement the techniques I've learned.

Regulating emotions is still a work in progress for me, but I've come a long way. By seeking help and being proactive in managing my emotions, I've regained control of my life and improved my relationships.

Introduction

Emotions are complex psychological states that encompass physiological responses, cognitive interpretations, and behavioural expressions. They play a crucial role in human experiences, influencing thoughts, decisions, and interactions. Common emotions include happiness, sadness, anger, fear, and surprise, each serving a unique function in how we respond to and navigate the world around us (Celeghin et al., 2017).

Emotional regulation refers to the processes through which individuals influence their emotions, how they experience them, and how they express them (McRae and Gross, 2020). This is like the body's internal thermostat for emotional reactions, whereby, if someone's thermostat under- or overreacts to a stimulus, the person can benefit from tools to improve their emotional regulation. Effective regulation of emotions involves recognising and managing both positive and negative emotions in a healthy manner. This skill is essential for maintaining mental health, fostering positive relationships, and achieving personal goals. By understanding and employing various strategies for emotional regulation, individuals can enhance their emotional well-being and overall quality of life.

Chapter Aims

This chapter will explore contemporary theory and practice around the following topics:

- What emotions are and how they can be influenced by different mental health presentations.

- Models of emotional regulation, including biosocial theory (Linehan, 1993), The Process Model (McRae and Gross, 2020), and Lazarus's cognitive-mediational theory (Lazarus, 1991).
- Tools to support you in equipping patients and service users to manage their emotions, which might also help you in regulating your own emotions in the context of sometimes stressful working and home lives.
- Understanding specialist interventions: Cognitive Behaviour Therapy (CBT), Dialectical Behaviour Therapy (DBT), Schema Therapy, and Acceptance and Commitment Therapy (ACT).

What Are Emotions?

Emotions are complex psychological states that encompass physiological arousal, cognitive appraisal, and expressive behaviours (Scherer, 2005). They serve as signals that guide our reactions to various situations and influence our thoughts, behaviours, and interactions with others. Emotions such as happiness, sadness, anger, fear, and surprise are fundamental to the human experience. They are felt in a multitude of ways. Happiness, for example, might manifest as a warm sensation accompanied by a smile, while anger might be experienced as a rush of adrenaline and an urge to confront a perceived threat. These emotional responses can be fleeting or enduring, and their intensity can vary based on the context and personal history (Gross and Thompson, 2007). The way emotions are experienced and expressed is also influenced by cultural, social, and personal factors, making them unique to each person. Understanding and regulating emotions is crucial for maintaining mental and emotional wellbeing.

Presentations Involving Emotional Distress

The way emotions reside in the body can present differently in different mental health diagnoses and presentations. These differences and similarities will now be explored.

Anxiety

Anxiety is a state of excessive worry, fear, or unease about real or perceived threats, often accompanied by physical symptoms such as increased heart rate, sweating, and tension. It can significantly impact a person's emotional experiences and regulation by heightening their sensitivity to stressors and amplifying emotional responses (Hofmann et al., 2012). An integrative review by Cisler et al. (2010) explored how the symptoms might present. For example, individuals with anxiety may find it difficult to manage their emotions, as the persistent state of alertness and worry can lead to rapid emotional escalation and difficulty returning to a calm state. This chronic activation of the body's stress response can interfere with cognitive processes, making it challenging to engage in effective strategies for emotional regulation, such as cognitive reappraisal or mindfulness. As a result, anxiety can create a cycle of emotional distress, further exacerbating the difficulty of managing and regulating emotions in various situations.

Depression

Depression is a serious mental health disorder characterised by persistent feelings of sadness, hopelessness, and a lack of interest or pleasure in activities once enjoyed (Beck et al., 2009). It often comes with physical symptoms such as changes in appetite, sleep disturbances, and fatigue. Depression can significantly influence a person's emotional experiences by amplifying negative emotions and diminishing the ability to feel positive emotions. This pervasive sense of despair can make it challenging to effectively manage and regulate emotions. Joorman and Stanton (2016) explain how individuals with depression may find themselves caught in a cycle of negative thoughts and feelings, making it difficult to engage in adaptive emotional regulation strategies like cognitive reappraisal or seeking social support. The overwhelming nature of depressive symptoms can lead to emotional numbness, where individuals feel detached or indifferent, further complicating their ability to connect with their emotions and manage them in healthy ways. Overall, depression can create substantial barriers to emotional regulation, affecting overall wellbeing and quality of life.

Borderline Personality Disorder

Borderline Personality Disorder (BPD, also known as Emotionally Unstable Personality Disorder or EUPD depending on which diagnostic manual is being used) is a mental health condition characterised by pervasive instability in moods, behaviour, self-image, and relationships. As explained by Linehan (1993), individuals diagnosed with BPD often experience intense emotions and have difficulty regulating them. This emotional volatility can lead to rapid mood swings, impulsive behaviours, and tumultuous relationships. The experience of emotions in BPD is marked by a heightened sensitivity to emotional stimuli and a slower return to emotional baseline, making it challenging to manage and regulate emotions effectively. Individuals with BPD may struggle with intense feelings of anger, sadness, and anxiety, which can lead to self-harm, substance abuse, or other maladaptive coping mechanisms.

Difficulty in regulating emotions can create a vicious cycle, where intense emotions lead to impulsive actions that, in turn, exacerbate emotional distress. This instability affects overall wellbeing and can significantly impair social, occupational, and personal functioning. Understanding and addressing the challenges of emotion regulation in BPD is crucial for improving the quality of life for those affected by this disorder.

Bipolar Disorder

This section would not be complete without considering bipolar disorder, because it is important to note that emotional dysregulation, which involves difficulty managing and responding to emotional experiences, is often mistaken for bipolar disorder. Emotional dysregulation can occur in various mental health conditions, but unlike bipolar disorder, which involves distinct episodes of mania and depression, emotional dysregulation is characterised by a more constant and pervasive difficulty in managing emotions. This distinction is crucial for accurate diagnosis and appropriate treatment, as the management strategies for bipolar disorder and emotional dysregulation can differ significantly.

The impact of emotional regulation and bipolar disorder has been explored by Kurtz et al. (2021) and De Prisco et al. (2023). Bipolar disorder is a mental health condition characterised by extreme mood swings occurring over a period of time, including episodes of mania (elevated mood, increased energy, and impulsive behaviour) and depression (persistent sadness, low energy, and loss of interest in activities). These mood swings can significantly impact a person's emotional experiences and regulation.

During manic episodes, individuals may feel euphoric, irritable, or excessively confident, leading to impulsive decisions and risky behaviours. Conversely, during depressive episodes, they may experience overwhelming sadness, hopelessness, and difficulty managing daily tasks. The rapid shifts between these emotional states can make it challenging for individuals with bipolar disorder to regulate their emotions effectively. They may struggle with maintaining stable relationships, holding down jobs, and managing their overall wellbeing.

Emotions – Shaped by Past Experiences, Trauma, and Biology

Emotions are significantly influenced by past experiences, which shape our emotional responses and perceptions (Mineka and Zinbarg, 2006). Positive experiences can lead to feelings of happiness, trust, and security, while negative experiences can result in feelings of fear, anger, or sadness. For example, a person who has experienced consistent support and affection in their upbringing may develop a sense of emotional stability and resilience. In contrast, someone who has faced neglect or abuse may have heightened sensitivity to stress and difficulty regulating emotions. Our past experiences create emotional templates that influence how we interpret and respond to new situations. This phenomenon is rooted in associative learning, where previous emotional responses become linked to specific triggers, shaping our future emotional reactions (Ochsner and Gross, 2008). Understanding the role of past experiences in shaping emotions is crucial for effective emotional regulation and mental health interventions.

Trauma can have a profound impact on emotional experiences and regulation. Traumatic events, such as physical or emotional abuse, accidents, or natural disasters, can lead to long-lasting emotional scars (McEwen, 2007). Trauma can cause heightened emotional reactivity, where individuals experience intense emotions in response to minor stressors. This emotional dysregulation is often a result of the brain's altered response to stress, as trauma affects the amygdala, hippocampus, and prefrontal cortex – each of which is a key area involved in processing emotions (Van Der Kolk, 2006). People who have experienced trauma may also develop maladaptive coping mechanisms, such as avoidance or numbing, to manage overwhelming emotions. These responses can interfere with healthy emotional regulation and increase the risk of mental health disorders, such as post-traumatic stress disorder (PTSD), anxiety, and depression. Addressing trauma through therapeutic interventions is essential for restoring emotional balance and wellbeing.

The biosocial theory, proposed by Crowell et al. (2009) and underpinning the work of Marsha Linehan (1993), states that emotional dysregulation arises from the interaction between biological predispositions and environmental influences. This theory is particularly relevant to understanding conditions like BPD. According to the biosocial theory, individuals with BPD have an innate emotional sensitivity and heightened emotional reactivity. This can be understood by thinking about individual differences in sensitivities to different washing powders or dietary sensitivities. When combined with an invalidating environment, where their emotional experiences are dismissed or punished, these individuals struggle to develop effective emotion regulation skills. An invalidating environment does not have to be abusive; it just needs to have a problem with fit. For example, a family of bakers whose child has a gluten intolerance is not abusive but is not a good fit. Similarly in the case of a kitten growing up in a family of lions! This theory highlights the importance of both biological factors, such as genetic and neurobiological vulnerabilities, and social factors, such as family dynamics and cultural influences, in shaping emotional regulation.

Process Model of Emotion Regulation

James Gross's Process Model of Emotion Regulation (Gross, 1998; Gross, 2002; Gross and Thompson, 2007) is a comprehensive framework that outlines how individuals can influence their emotional experiences at different stages of the emotion-generative process. The model identifies five key stages: situation selection, situation modification, attentional deployment, cognitive change, and response modulation. Each stage offers unique opportunities for intervention to regulate emotions effectively.

Situation Selection

This involves choosing which situations to enter or avoid, based on their potential emotional impact. By proactively selecting situations that are likely to elicit positive emotions and avoiding those that may trigger negative emotions, individuals can manage their emotional experiences more effectively. For example, someone who feels anxious in crowded places might choose to shop during off-peak hours to minimise stress.

Situation Modification

This refers to the ways individuals can modify situations they are in to influence their emotional response. This might involve changing aspects of the environment or altering their behaviour to make the situation more manageable. For instance, if attending a social event is unavoidable, a person could choose to stay close to a supportive friend or engage in activities that reduce anxiety.

Attentional Deployment

This involves the person directing their focus within a given situation to regulate emotions. Techniques such as distraction, concentration, or mindfulness can help individuals manage their emotional responses. For example, focusing on a calming aspect of the environment or engaging in a mentally absorbing task can help reduce feelings of distress.

Cognitive Change

This involves a person altering thoughts or appraisals about a situation to change its emotional impact. This can be achieved through cognitive reappraisal, where individuals reinterpret the meaning of an event to elicit a more positive emotional response. For example, viewing a challenging task as an opportunity for growth rather than a threat can reduce anxiety and increase motivation.

Response Modulation

Response modulation occurs after an emotion has been fully generated and involves strategies to influence the physiological, experiential, or behavioural aspects of the emotional response. Techniques such as deep breathing, progressive muscle relaxation, or expressive suppression can help individuals manage their emotional reactions. For instance, taking deep breaths to calm oneself during a stressful situation can help reduce physiological arousal and promote emotional regulation.

Cognitive-Mediational Theory

Richard Lazarus's cognitive-mediational theory of emotion (Lazarus, 1991; Smith and Lazarus, 1993; Folkman, 2013) emphasises the role of cognitive appraisal in the emotional response process. According to this theory, emotions are not just automatic reactions to events but are shaped by how individuals interpret or evaluate those events. The theory posits that our thoughts mediate, or come between, the event and our emotional response, highlighting the importance of cognitive processes in shaping emotions.

The first stage in Lazarus's cognitive-mediational theory is primary appraisal, where individuals assess whether a situation is relevant to their wellbeing. During this stage, people evaluate the significance of an event by asking questions like, "Is this situation harmful?" or "Does this affect me personally?" If the event is deemed significant or poses a threat, an emotional response begins to form. For example, if someone sees a car speeding towards them, their primary appraisal might be, "This is dangerous!" leading to feelings of fear.

The second stage is secondary appraisal, where individuals evaluate their ability to cope with the situation. During this stage, people assess their resources and options for managing the event by asking questions like, "What can I do about this?" or "Do I have the resources to handle it?" If individuals believe they can cope with the situation, their emotional response may be less intense. Conversely, if they feel helpless, the emotional reaction can become stronger. For example, if someone sees an escape route and thinks, "I can jump out of the way", their fear may reduce. However, if they feel trapped, the fear is very likely to intensify.

Lazarus's cognitive-mediational theory also provides insight into the relationship between stress and emotion. According to Lazarus, stress arises from the ways individuals appraise situations as threatening or challenging as well as their perceived ability to cope with them. If people believe an event is a threat and that they lack the resources to handle it, they experience stress. However, if they believe they can manage the situation, the stress is reduced. This understanding is crucial for managing stress, as it suggests that changing how we think about a situation can help us manage our emotional responses more effectively.

Emotions as a Form of Communication

Emotions are fundamental to human communication, serving as innate signals that convey important information about our internal states and intentions (Dennison, 2024). From an evolutionary perspective, emotions have developed as adaptive responses to environmental challenges, helping individuals navigate social interactions and ensure survival. For example, facial expressions indicating emotions such as fear, anger, and happiness are universally recognised across cultures, indicating that these emotional expressions are biologically hardwired and serve as a universal language (Keltner and Ekman, 2008). These expressions provide critical cues to others about potential threats, social bonds, and cooperative behaviours, facilitating effective communication and social cohesion.

Primary emotions, such as joy, distress, anger, fear, surprise, and disgust, are considered innate because they are experienced by everyone, regardless of cultural and social influences, and appear rapidly in response to external stimuli (Bell and Farmer, 2025). These emotions are often accompanied by distinct facial expressions and physiological changes that are easily recognised by others. For instance, a smile indicates happiness and can foster social bonding, while a frown or a look of fear can signal distress and elicit support from others. The ability to express and interpret these primary emotions is crucial for effective interpersonal communication, as it allows individuals to respond appropriately to the emotional states of others and navigate social interactions smoothly and more effectively.

While the experience of these primary emotions is innate, the expression and interpretation of emotions is also shaped by socialisation and cultural norms. From a young age, individuals learn to recognise and respond to the emotional cues of others through social interactions (de Melo et al., 2021). This process of socialisation helps individuals develop emotional intelligence, which is the ability to understand and manage our emotions as well as the emotions of others (D'Amico and Geraci, 2023). Emotional intelligence is essential for building and maintaining healthy relationships, as it enables individuals to effectively communicate feelings, as well as empathise with others. Cultural norms and display rules also influence how emotions are expressed and perceived, highlighting the interplay between biological and social factors in emotional communication (Mancini et al., 2022).

Tools for Now: Small Changes That Can Make a Big Difference

In this section, a number of techniques you can use are presented (for example, validation) as well as ones that you can teach patients and service users (such as grounding techniques). Each of these techniques could also be useful for healthcare practitioners when reflecting on practice, as well as in managing any difficult emotions that arise through their work or everyday life.

Validation

Understanding emotions as innate methods of communication underscores the importance of validation by healthcare professionals in mental health care. Validation involves recognising and affirming the emotional experiences of patients and service users as legitimate and understandable, which is crucial for effective therapeutic relationships (Wasson Simpson et al., 2021). When healthcare practitioners validate a person's emotions, they acknowledge that individual's internal state and their efforts to communicate distress, needs, or desires. This recognition fosters a sense of trust and safety, encouraging patients to share their experiences more freely.

Validation helps reduce feelings of isolation and shame, as patients feel heard and understood. It also promotes emotional regulation by providing a supportive environment where patients can process and manage their emotions more effectively. By validating emotions, healthcare professionals facilitate better communication, enhance the therapeutic alliance, and support the patient's journey towards emotional healing and enhanced wellbeing.

The "What" Skill

The "What" skill in DBT is a core mindfulness practice that involves three key actions: observing, describing, and participating (Linehan, 2015). Observing means noticing your thoughts, feelings, and sensations without judgement. Describing involves putting words to your experiences, accurately labelling what you observe. Participating means fully engaging in the present moment and taking part in activities with awareness. These skills are crucial for emotional regulation as they help individuals become more aware of their emotional states and reactions. By observing and describing emotions without judgement, individuals can gain a clearer understanding of their emotional triggers and patterns. This awareness allows people to respond to emotions more effectively, rather than reacting impulsively. Participating in the present moment helps individuals stay grounded and reduces the intensity of negative emotions.

The "How" Skill

The "How" skill in DBT complements the "What" skill by focusing on the quality of mindfulness practice (Linehan, 2015). It includes three key components of practice: non-judgementally, one-mindfully, and effectively. Practising non-judgementally means observing and describing emotions without labelling them as "good" or "bad." This helps reduce emotional intensity and promotes acceptance of emotional experiences. One-mindfully involves focusing on one thing at a time, which helps individuals stay present and fully engage in the moment. This can reduce feelings of overwhelm and increase emotional clarity. Effectively means doing what works in each situation, which involves being flexible and using skills that are appropriate for the context. By practising the "How" skill, individuals can approach their emotions with a mindful and balanced attitude, enhancing the ability to regulate emotions effectively. This mindful approach supports emotional regulation by promoting acceptance, focus, and adaptive responses to emotional challenges.

Distress Tolerance

Distress tolerance is a crucial component of DBT that focuses on helping individuals manage and endure intense emotional pain without resorting to impulsive or harmful behaviours (Linehan, 2015). It involves developing skills to tolerate and survive crises, such as distraction techniques, self-soothing methods, and grounding exercises. Distress tolerance plays a vital role in emotional regulation by providing individuals with practical tools to cope with overwhelming emotions in the short term. By effectively tolerating distress, individuals can prevent emotional escalation, reduce impulsive reactions, and create a sense of stability. This allows them to approach their emotions more mindfully and regulate them in healthier ways, ultimately promoting emotional wellbeing and resilience (Heiland and Veilleux, 2024).

The "TIPP" Skills

The "TIPP" skills in DBT is a distress tolerance technique designed to help individuals manage intense emotions and reduce emotional arousal quickly (Linehan, 2015). "TIPP" stands for Temperature, Intense exercise, Paced breathing, and Progressive muscle relaxation. Each component targets the body's physiological response to stress, promoting emotional regulation.

Temperature

This involves using cold temperatures to bring down the body's arousal level. For example, holding ice, splashing cold water on the face, or placing a cold pack on the back of the neck can activate the body's dive reflex, which slows the heart rate and calms the nervous system. This helps reduce the intensity of overwhelming emotions. Due to this skill simulating the dive reflex and reducing the heart rate, those with heart conditions, blood pressure concerns, those on medication that can reduce blood pressure, those with cold sensitivity, or an eating disorder, should consult with their health care professional before using this skill.

Intense Exercise

Engaging in short bursts of intense physical activity, such as running, jumping jacks, or dancing, can help burn off excess energy and reduce emotional distress. Exercise releases endorphins, which are natural mood elevators, and helps shift focus away from distressing thoughts and feelings.

Paced Breathing

This involves slowing down the breath to calm the body's stress response. Techniques such as diaphragmatic breathing, where one inhales deeply through the nose, holds the breath for a few seconds, and then exhales slowly through the mouth, can help regulate emotions by promoting relaxation and reducing anxiety.

Progressive Muscle Relaxation

This technique involves systematically tensing and then relaxing different muscle groups in the body. By focusing on the physical sensations of tension and relaxation, individuals can release built-up stress and promote a sense of calm. This practice helps interrupt the cycle of emotional escalation and fosters emotional regulation.

Grounding Techniques

Grounding is a set of techniques used to help individuals bring their focus onto the present moment, often by engaging their senses or redirecting their thoughts. It is particularly useful for managing intense emotions, anxiety, and stress by reducing the impact of distressing thoughts and feelings (Keptner et al., 2021). Grounding techniques help individuals become more aware of their surroundings and their bodies, which can provide a sense of stability and control. This awareness aids in emotional regulation by interrupting the cycle of emotional escalation and promoting a sense of calm. By staying connected to the present moment, grounding techniques enable individuals to better manage their emotional responses and maintain emotional balance.

One grounding technique is the 5-4-3-2-1 method, which helps individuals anchor themselves in the present moment by engaging their senses. This technique is particularly effective for managing anxiety, stress, and overwhelming emotions. The technique involves identifying and focusing on sensory experiences to bring attention back to the present moment. The following explanation illustrates how it works:

Identify and pay attention to each of the following, saying them out loud if you are in an appropriate setting to do so:

5 **Things You Can See**: Look around and name five things you can see. This could be anything in your immediate environment, such as a clock on the wall, a plant, or a piece of furniture.

4   **Things You Can Feel**: Focus on four things you can physically feel. This might include the texture of your clothing, the sensation of your feet on the ground, or the feeling of a chair against your back.

3   **Things You Can Hear**: Listen carefully and identify three things you can hear. This could be the sound of birds chirping, the hum of the air conditioning, or distant traffic noise.

2   **Things You Can Smell**: Notice two things you can smell. This might be the scent of your perfume, the aroma of food, or the smell of fresh air.

1   **Thing You Can Taste**: Pay attention to one thing you can taste. This could be the taste of gum, a sip of water, or the lingering flavour of a meal.

By systematically engaging each of the five senses, the 5-4-3-2-1 technique helps individuals to shift their focus away from distressing thoughts and reconnect with the present moment.

"Check the Facts"

The "What" and the "How" skills previously discussed can be used in conjunction with a skill to help people check if their thoughts are judgements or not. "Check the Facts" is a cognitive-behavioural technique often used in DBT to help individuals challenge and reframe distorted or inaccurate thoughts and beliefs (Linehan, 2015). The process involves examining the evidence for and against a particular thought or belief to determine its accuracy. By identifying cognitive distortions, such as catastrophising or overgeneralising, individuals can replace unhelpful thoughts with more balanced and realistic ones. Encouraging the person to check the facts can reduce the intensity of negative emotions, such as anxiety or anger, so that a more rational and grounded perspective can be adopted. This helps in managing emotional responses more effectively and promotes overall mental wellbeing.

"Opposite Action"

"Opposite action" is a cognitive-behavioural technique often used in DBT to help individuals change their emotional responses by engaging in behaviours that are opposite to their current emotional urges (Linehan,

2015). When experiencing intense emotions, individuals may have the urge to act in ways that reinforce those emotions, such as avoiding social situations when feeling anxious or lashing out when feeling angry. Opposite action involves identifying the emotional urge and intentionally choosing to engage in behaviours that counteract that urge. This can be used in the moment as a de-escalation strategy coached by the professional or as a goal planning strategy. In the moment, if a healthcare practitioner notices that a person appears angry and they are tense and adopting a large body posture with fast breathing and a loud voice, they can coach and model opposite behaviours, getting the person to reduce their body posture, lower their voice, and slow their breathing. In longer-term goal planning, if someone feels the urge to isolate themselves due to sadness, they might choose to reach out to a friend or to engage in a social activity instead. This technique is crucial for emotional regulation, as it helps break the cycle of negative emotions and promotes healthier, more adaptive responses.

Acceptance

Acceptance is a key component of many therapeutic approaches, including Acceptance and Commitment Therapy (ACT). It involves acknowledging and embracing one's emotions, thoughts, and experiences without attempting to change, suppress, or judge them (Wojnarowska et al., 2020). By adopting an open and non-judgemental attitude towards emotions, individuals can reduce the struggle against negative feelings and create space for more adaptive responses. Acceptance plays a crucial role in emotional regulation by allowing individuals to experience emotions fully without being overwhelmed by them. This approach helps individuals develop greater emotional resilience and flexibility, enabling them to navigate challenging situations more effectively. Acceptance fosters a sense of self-compassion and reduces the impact of negative emotions on overall wellbeing. As a relatively trivial example, imagine how you would feel on returning home from work to find that your housemate has eaten the chocolate bar you had been looking forward to all day. You could well experience distress in this situation. Being cross with your housemate, thinking about the unfairness of the situation, and wishing they hadn't taken your treat adds additional layers of emotional distress to the initial distress of your treat being gone, whereas accepting that they have taken it is likely to alleviate some of the distress.

Managing and Regulating Emotions: Understanding Specialist Interventions

Cognitive-Behavioural Therapy (CBT)

A widely used, evidence-based psychotherapeutic approach, CBT focuses on identifying and modifying negative thought patterns and behaviours to improve emotional regulation and overall mental health (Nezu and Nezu, 2016). CBT is grounded in the concept that our thoughts, feelings, and behaviours are interconnected, and that changing maladaptive thoughts can lead to changes in emotions and behaviours. As a specialist intervention for emotional regulation, CBT helps individuals develop skills to recognise and challenge cognitive distortions, such as catastrophising or overgeneralising, and to replace them with more balanced and realistic thoughts (Mahali et al., 2020). Techniques such as cognitive restructuring, behavioural activation, and exposure therapy are commonly used in CBT to address emotional dysregulation. By learning to manage their thoughts and behaviours more effectively, individuals can reduce the intensity and frequency of negative emotions, enhance emotional resilience, and improve their overall wellbeing.

Dialectical Behaviour Therapy

DBT is a specialised form of CBT developed by psychologist Marsha Linehan in the late 1980s (Linehan, 1993, 2015). Initially designed to treat individuals with BPD, DBT has since been adapted to address a wide range of emotional and behavioural challenges. DBT combines principles of acceptance and change, helping individuals develop skills to manage intense emotions, reduce self-destructive behaviours, and improve relationships.

This therapy consists of four main components: mindfulness, distress tolerance, emotion regulation, and interpersonal effectiveness. Emotion regulation skills in DBT teach individuals to understand and manage their emotions effectively, reducing emotional vulnerability and fostering positive emotional experiences. By integrating these skills into daily life, individuals can achieve greater emotional stability and resilience.

Schema Therapy

Developed by Jeffrey Young in the 1990s, this integrative therapeutic approach combines elements of CBT, attachment theory and psychodynamic therapy, with experiential techniques (Young, 1990). It is designed to treat individuals with deep-rooted emotional patterns, which can be formed in response to unmet emotional needs during childhood.

In the context of Schema Therapy, a schema refers to a deep-seated pattern or theme of thoughts, feelings, and behaviours that develops during childhood and continues to influence an individual's life in adulthood (Young, 1990). These schemas are often formed in response to unmet emotional needs or adverse experiences and become ingrained as ways of understanding and interacting with the world. Schemas can be both positive and negative, but in therapy, the focus is typically on early maladaptive schemas that lead to dysfunctional behaviours and emotional distress.

Early maladaptive schemas are categorised into different domains based on the core emotional needs they represent, such as the need for safety, connection, autonomy, and self-esteem. For example, a schema of "abandonment" may develop in individuals who experienced instability or loss in their early relationships, leading to a persistent fear of being left alone. Other common schemas include "defectiveness," where individuals feel inherently flawed, and "unrelenting standards," where individuals believe they must meet impossibly high expectations to gain approval.

Schema Therapy aims to help individuals identify, understand, and change these maladaptive schemas. Through various techniques, such as cognitive restructuring, experiential exercises, and limited reparenting, therapists work with clients to challenge and heal these deep-rooted patterns, fostering healthier ways of thinking, feeling, and behaving. The therapy focuses on identifying and changing early maladaptive schemas and coping styles that contribute to emotional dysregulation (Dadomo et al., 2016). By addressing the core emotional themes and using techniques such as imagery rescripting, limited reparenting, and chair work, Schema Therapy helps individuals develop healthier emotional responses and improve emotional regulation. This approach is particularly effective for individuals with personality disorders, chronic depression, and trauma.

Acceptance and Commitment Therapy (ACT)

This is a form of CBT that emphasises psychological flexibility through acceptance, mindfulness, and values-driven action. Developed by Steven Hayes in the 1980s, ACT encourages individuals to accept their thoughts and feelings rather than trying to control or avoid them (Hayes, 1987). The core processes of ACT include acceptance, cognitive defusion, being present, self-as-context, values, and committed action. These processes help individuals develop a more adaptive relationship with their internal experiences, allowing them to live a meaningful life aligned with their values.

As a therapy to enhance emotional regulation, ACT promotes the idea that struggling with or avoiding negative emotions often exacerbates emotional distress (Powers et al., 2009). Instead, ACT teaches individuals to accept their emotions as a natural part of the human experience and to observe them without judgement. By practising mindfulness and cognitive defusion, individuals can reduce the impact of distressing thoughts and emotions, enhancing their ability to respond to challenging situations with clarity and calm. This approach fosters emotional resilience and flexibility, enabling individuals to navigate life's stressors more effectively and to maintain emotional wellbeing.

Summary of Learning Points

This chapter has explored the following theoretical and practical approaches to emotional regulation:

- What emotions are and how they can present in different mental health diagnoses, particularly in relation to anxiety, depression, bipolar disorder and borderline personality disorder, each of which has emotional features as part of their cluster of symptoms.
- The impact of trauma on emotions and the biosocial model have been considered, along with a range of models and theories around emotional regulation and dysregulation. These include The Process Model of emotional regulation and the cognitive-mediational theory of emotion.
- A wealth of tools that can be used to support individuals in the moment are presented, with an emphasis on the importance of validation, and the usefulness of a range of DBT skills, which can be adopted and used to

support patients and service users, as well as being used by practitioners who are experiencing heightened emotions in the context of their work, or personal lives.

- Interventions for emotional dysregulation, for which patients and service users may be referred to specialist services, include CBT, DBT, Schema Therapy, and ACT.

Questions for Reflection and Discussion

1. How can you integrate mindfulness practices, such as observing, describing, and participating, into your daily routine to enhance your own emotional regulation?

2. Identify scenarios where you might have noticed features of your own or your patients' and service user's emotions, considering how the insights gained by reading this chapter could change your response, in the moment, to such emotions.

3. How could you use "opposite action" to support the regulation of your own emotions, as well as encourage this approach with patients and service users?

4. How can you challenge and reframe negative thoughts with patients and service users (for example, through "Check the Facts" or acceptance techniques) to support them in improving their emotional responses and overall wellbeing?

5. Identify examples of how early maladaptive schemas might influence emotional reactions. How can we work towards healing such schemas to improve emotional regulation and relationships?

Recommended Follow-up Reading

Brillon, P., Dewar, M., Lapointe, V., Paradis, A. and Philippe, F.L. (2025). Emotion regulation and compassion fatigue in mental health professionals in a context of stress: A longitudinal study. *PloS Mental Health*. 2(2): e0000187: 1–14.

Centre for Clinical Interventions (2019). Looking after yourself: Depression. Available online at: https://www.cci.health.wa.gov.au/Resources/Looking-After-Yourself/Depression. [Accessed 20th August 2025].

Linehan, M.M. (2015). *DBT Skills Training Manual*. (2nd ed). New York: Guilford Press.

Pálfi, K., Major, J., Horváth-Sarródi, A., Deák, A., Fehér, G. and Gács, B. (2024). Adaptive emotion regulation might prevent burnout in emergency healthcare professionals: An exploratory study. *BMC Public Health*. 24(1): 1–10.

Salvarani, V., Rampoldi, G., Ardenghi, S., Bani, M., Blasi, P., Ausili, D., Di Mauro, S. and Strepparava, M.G. (2019). Protecting emergency room nurses from burnout: The role of dispositional mindfulness, emotion regulation and empathy. *Journal of Nursing Management*. 27(4): 765–774.

References

Beck, A.T. and Alford, B.A. (2009). *Depression: Causes and Treatment*. (2nd ed). Philadelphia: University of Pennsylvania Press.

Bell, B. and Farmer, D. (2025). Oral/interpersonal communications. Available online at: https://wtcs.pressbooks.pub/oralinterpersonalcomm/. [Accessed 14th August 2025].

Celeghin, A., Diano, M., Bagnis, A., Viola, M. and Tamietto, M. (2017). Basic emotions in human neuroscience: Neuroimaging and beyond. *Frontiers in Psychology*. 8, Article 1432: 1–13.

Cisler, J.M., Olantunji, B.O., Feldner, M.T. and Forsyth, J.P. (2010). Emotional regulation and the anxiety disorders: An integrative review. *Journal of Psychopathology and Behavioral Assessment*. 32: 68–82.

Crowell, S.E., Beauchaine, T.P. and Linehan, M.M. (2009). A biosocial developmental model of borderline personality: Elaborating and extending Linehan's theory. *Psychological Bulletin*. 135(3): 495–510.

Dadomo, H., Grecucci, A., Giardini, I., Ugolini, E., Carmelita, A. and Panzeri, M. (2016). Schema therapy for emotional dysregulation: Theoretical implication and clinical applications. *Frontiers in Psychology*. 7, Article 1987: 1–17.

D'Amico, A. and Geraci, A. (2023). Beyond emotional intelligence: The new construct of meta-emotional intelligence. *Frontiers in Psychology*. 14: 1–12.

de Melo, C.M., Terada, K. and Santos, F.C. (2021). Emotion expressions shape human social norms and reputations. *ISCIENCE*. 24(3): 1–8.

Dennison, J. (2024). Emotions: Functions and significance for attitudes, behaviour, and communication. *Migration Studies*. 12(1): 1–20.

De Prisco, M., Oliva, V., Fico, G., Radua, J., Grande, I., Roberto, N., Anmella, G., Hidalgo-Mazzei, D., Fornaro, M. and de Bartolomeis, A. (2023). Emotion dysregulation in bipolar disorder compared to other mental illnesses: A systematic review and meta-analysis. *Psychological Medicine*. 53(16): 7484–7503.

Folkman, S. (2013). *Stress: Appraisal and coping*. In M.D. Gellman and J.R. Turner (Eds.), *Encyclopedia of Behavioral Medicine*. New York: Springer, pp. 1913–1915.

Gross, J.J. (1998). The emerging field of emotion regulation: An integrative review. *Review of General Psychology*. 2(3): 271–299.

Gross, J.J. (2002). Emotion regulation: Affective, cognitive, and social consequences. *Psychophysiology*. 39(3): 281–291.

Gross, J.J. and Thompson, R.A. (2007). Emotion regulation: Conceptual foundations. In J.J. Gross (Ed.), *Handbook of Emotion Regulation*. New York: Guilford Press, pp. 3–24.

Hayes, S.C. (1987). A contextual approach to therapeutic change: The concept of cognitive distancing. *The Behavior Analyst*. 10(1): 27–44.

Heiland, A.M. and Veilleux, J.C. (2024). Reductions in distress intolerance via intervention: A review. *Cognitive Therapy and Research*. 48: 833–853.

Hofmann, S.G., Sawyer, A.T., Fang, A. and Asnaani, A. (2012). Emotion dysregulation model of mood and anxiety disorders. *Depression and Anxiety*. 29: 409–416.

Joorman, J. and Stanton, C.H. (2016). Examining emotion regulation in depression: A review and future directions. *Behaviour Research and Therapy*. 86: 35–49.

Keltner, D. and Ekman, P. (2008). *Facial expression of emotion*. In M. Lewis, J.M. Haviland-Jones and L.F. Barrett (Eds.), *Handbook of Emotions* (3rd ed). New York: Guilford Press, pp. 211–234.

Keptner, K.M., Fitzgibbon, C. and O'Sullivan, J. (2021). Effectiveness of anxiety reduction interventions on test anxiety: A comparison of four techniques incorporating sensory modulation. *British Journal of Occupational Therapy*. 84(5): 289–297.

Kurtz, M., Mohring, P., Forster, K., Bauer, M. and Kanske, P. (2021). Deficits in explicit emotion regulation in bipolar disorder: A systematic review. *International Journal of Bipolar Disorders*. 9(1): 1–23.

Lazarus, R.S. (1991). *Emotion and Adaption*. New York: Oxford University Press.

Linehan, M. (1993). *Cognitive-Behavioural Treatment for Borderline Personality Disorder*. New York: Guilford Press.

Linehan, M. (2015). *DBT Skills Training Manual*. (2nd ed). New York: Guilford Press.

Mahali, S.C., Beshai, S., Feeney, J.R. and Mishra, S. (2020). Associations of negative cognitions, emotional regulation, and depression symptoms across four continents: International support for the cognitive model of depression. *BMC Psychiatry*. 20(18): 1–12.

Mancini, G., Biolcati, R., Joseph, D., Tromboni, E. and Andrei, F. (2022). Editorial: Emotional intelligence: Current research and future perspectives on mental health and individual differences. *Frontiers in Psychology*. 13: 1–3.

McEwen, B.S. (2007). Physiology and neurobiology of stress and adaptation: Central role of the brain. *Physiological Reviews*. 87(3): 799–1082.

McRae, K. and Gross, J.J. (2020). Emotional regulation. *Emotion*. 20(1): 1–9.

Mineka, S. and Zinbarg, R. (2006). A contemporary learning theory perspective on the etiology of anxiety disorders: It's not what you thought it was. *American Psychologist*. 61(1): 10–26.

Nezu, C.M. and Nezu, A.M. (2016). *The Oxford Handbook of Cognitive and Behavioural Therapies*. Oxford: Oxford University Press.

Ochsner, K.N. and Gross, J.J. (2008). Cognitive emotion regulation: Insights from social cognitive and affective neuroscience. *Current Directions in Psychological Science*. 17(2): 153–158.

Powers, M.B., Vörding, M.B.Z.V.S. and Emmelkamp, P.M.G. (2009). Acceptance and commitment therapy: A meta-analytic review. *Psychotherapy and Psychosomatics*. 78(2): 73–80.

Scherer, K.R. (2005). What are emotions? And how can they be measured? *Social Science Information*. 44(4): 695–729.

Smith, C.A. and Lazarus, R.S. (1993). Appraisal components, core relational themes, and the emotions. *Cognition and Emotion*. 7(3–4): 233–269.

Van Der Kolk, B.A. (2006). Clinical implications of neuroscience esearch in PTSD. *Annals of the New York Academy of Sciences*. 1071: 277–293.

Wasson Simpson, K.S., Gallagher, A., Ronis, S.T., Miller, D.A.A. and Tilexzek, K.C. (2021). Youths' perceived impact of invalidation and validation on their mental health treatment journeys. *Administration and Policy in Mental Health and Mental Health Services Research*. 49: 476–489.

Wojnarowska, A., Kobylinska, D. and Lewczuk, K. (2020). Acceptance as an emotion regulation strategy in experimental psychological research: What we know and how we can improve that knowledge. *Frontiers in Psychology*. 11, Article 242: 1–5.

Young, J.E. (1990). *Cognitive Therapy for Personality Disorders: A Schema-Focused Approach*. Sarasota, FL: Professional Resource Exchange.

Stress and Distress

Actions and Reactions

Louise Cherrill

Case Study

Alice's Story

I have been struggling with anxiety and depression for several years. Despite trying various self-help techniques and leaning on my support system, symptoms have persisted and have begun to affect my daily life. I was determined to seek professional help, so decided to visit my General Practitioner (GP) to discuss my concerns about my mental health.

During the initial consultation, I felt really nervous but also quite hopeful. As I started to share my feelings and experiences, the GP seemed attentive and empathic. However, as the conversation progressed, the GP's responses seemed to become somewhat dismissive, with him suggesting that I take medication without having explored my experiences and underlying issues as thoroughly as I thought he should. This lack of understanding left me feeling unheard and invalidated.

I started feeling increasingly distressed and could feel my whole demeanour changing. Without meaning for it to happen, my voice grew louder, and I began gesturing in a more animated way. I was trying to express the seriousness of my struggles, but my heightened emotional state made it difficult for me to properly articulate my thoughts and as the appointment went on, I felt increasingly misunderstood. In fact, the GP, physically backed off a bit, as though he perceived my

DOI: 10.4324/9781003635611-4

actions and what I was saying as threatening. He seemed to become more defensive and less compassionate.

This misinterpretation of what I wanted to express exacerbated my distress still further, to the point where I banged my fists on my lap. I felt trapped in a cycle where the more I tried to communicate my pain the greater the misunderstanding and judgement that came back at me. In a final effort to make my point, with my frustration boiling over, I banged my clenched fist on the table between me and the doctor. I then stood up to leave, my voice still rising and with tears rolling down my face all the time. I left the room at that point, but my final outburst left me feeling really unsettled and embarrassed, as well as out of control. I can imagine that the doctor was equally unsettled, and that I had made a really bad impression on him.

Afterwards, I felt both shame and anger. I knew the way I had acted could well have seemed aggressive, but my distress had been a cry for help, and that hadn't seemed to have been properly recognised. The experience left me feeling totally isolated and unsure of where I could turn for support.

Introduction

Stress is an inherent part of the human experience, affecting everyone at some point in their lives. While it can carry negative connotations, it is a complex phenomenon, having impacts on our wellbeing, which could be both beneficial and detrimental. Understanding stress requires a multifaceted approach, encompassing biological, social, and psychological perspectives.

Chapter Aims

This chapter will focus on stress and distress, including information and ideas related to:

- Biological understandings of acute and chronic stress.
- Psychological models for understanding stress.

- Social models for understanding stress.
- Tools you can use in the moment to support people who are stressed, distressed, or who may appear angry or agitated.
- Specialist interventions for managing stress, distress, and expressions of agitation and anger.

Biological Understandings of Stress

From a biological standpoint, stress triggers a cascade of physiological responses aimed at helping the body cope with perceived threats. Key systems, such as the hypothalamic-pituitary-adrenal (HPA) axis and the sympathomedullary (SAM) pathway, facilitate the release of stress hormones like cortisol and adrenaline (Ravi et al., 2021). These hormones prepare the body for immediate action, enhancing survival in short-term situations where some kind of threat is posed. However, chronic activation of these systems can lead to adverse health outcomes, including cardiovascular disease, immune system suppression, diabetes, cancer, and mental health disorders (Ravi et al., 2021).

Understanding the SAM Pathway: The Body's Immediate Stress Response

Imagine that you are driving, when suddenly a car swerves in front of you. Your heart pounds, your palms get sweaty, and you feel an instant jolt of energy. This is your body's immediate stress response, often referred to as the fight-or-flight response, and at the core of this response is the SAM pathway (Sarmiento et al., 2024).

The SAM pathway involves two main components: the sympathetic nervous system (SNS) and the adrenal medulla. The SNS is the part of the nervous system responsible for preparing the body to handle stressful situations. When a threat is perceived, the SNS sends signals throughout the body to get ready for quick action, leading to an increased heart rate, expanded airways to increase oxygen intake, and diverting blood flow to essential muscles (Sarmiento et al., 2024). The adrenal medulla is located at the top of the kidneys and works closely with the SNS. When activated, it releases adrenaline (also known as epinephrine) into the bloodstream. Adrenaline is a powerful hormone that boosts energy levels, sharpens focus, and primes the body to either confront the threat or flee from it. It is this combination of SNS activation and adrenaline release that causes the fight-or-flight response, which is the body's way of making sure it is physically prepared to respond to immediate danger (McCarty, 2016). Once the threat passes, the parasympathetic nervous system (PNS) takes over, working to calm down the body by slowing heart and respiration rates and promoting relaxation (McCarty, 2016).

The SAM pathway is crucial for survival, but it is designed for short bursts of activity. When faced with constant stress, this system can remain overactive, leading to wear and tear on the body and contributing to health issues like high blood pressure and heart disease (Ravi et al., 2021). However, the SAM pathway is not the only pathway activated by stress; the HPA axis is a slower pathway that is activated in response to chronic stress.

Understanding the HPA Axis: Responding to Sustained Stress

When a stressor continues beyond the initial fight-or-flight response, the HPA axis activates. An example might be in a situation where you are caring for someone you love, who is living with a chronic illness. Day after day, you need to juggle the responsibilities of the care role, worrying about their wellbeing, as well as your own, frequently struggling with emotional and physical exhaustion. The prolonged stress will take a toll. Unlike the immediate fight-or-flight surge of the SAM pathway, the HPA axis gradually releases cortisol, helping the body to endure ongoing demands. The HPA axis is a complex system involving three key players: the hypothalamus, the pituitary gland, and the adrenal glands (Sarmiento et al., 2024). Table 3.1 shows the role of each part of the HPA axis in facilitating the prolonged stress response.

Table 3.1 The Role of the HPA Axis in Responding to Prolonged Stress

Anatomical structure	Function in responding to prolonged stress
Hypothalamus (the command centre)	• Perceives the threat • Sends corticotropin-releasing hormone (CRH)
Pituitary gland (the "master gland")	• Receives the CRH and releases adrenocorticotropic hormone (ACTH) into the bloodstream
Adrenal glands (on top of the kidneys)	• Detect ACTH and produce cortisol. • Cortisol increases blood sugar and suppresses systems not needed for immediate survival (e.g. digestive and immune systems)

When the immediate threat passes, the hypothalamus stops releasing corticotropin-releasing hormone (CRH), leading to a decrease in adrenocorticotropic hormone (ACTH) and cortisol levels, thus returning the body to its resting state. The HPA axis is essential for dealing with short-term stress, but chronic stress can keep this system activated, potentially leading to health problems such as anxiety and depression, as well as cardiovascular issues (Ravi et al., 2021).

How the HPA and SAM Systems Work Together

Firstly, the pathways use sequential activation, with the SAM pathway acting first to produce an immediate response and the HPA axis coming into play if the stressor persists. Secondly, the pathways have complementary roles, whereby adrenaline (from the SAM pathway) handles immediate, short-term stress, while cortisol (from the HPA axis) manages longer-term stress, ensuring the body can sustain its state of alert. Lastly, the pathways use regulation and feedback mechanisms. When cortisol levels rise, the pathways signal the hypothalamus and pituitary gland to reduce CRH and ACTH production, thus preventing excessive stress responses.

While biological models such as the HPA axis and SAM pathway explain the physiological mechanisms behind stress, they do not operate in isolation. Stress is not only a biological process but is significantly shaped by social and environmental factors. Individual experiences, societal expectations, and cultural influences each play a role in how stress is perceived, managed, and exacerbated.

Social Understandings of Stress

Moving beyond the physiological framework, this section explores the social dimensions of stress, examining how relationships, socioeconomic status, and societal pressures contribute to stress responses in everyday life. Social dimensions of stress concern how our interactions and relationships influence our stress levels. As explained in Cohen and Willis's (1985) seminal work, social support networks, cultural norms, and socioeconomic status each play pivotal roles in shaping our stress experiences. Strong social connections can buffer the impact of stress, providing emotional support and practical assistance. Conversely, social isolation or negative social interactions can exacerbate stress, contributing to feelings of loneliness and helplessness.

Social Impacts on Experiences of Stress

Social Stress Theories highlight that our stress experiences are deeply influenced by our social environment, such that perception of stress is deeper than our internal thoughts or immediate circumstances. They also take into consideration the broader social context in which we live. Surachman and Almeida (2018) explore how social structures and hierarchies play a significant role in creating stress. Factors like socioeconomic status, race, gender, and employment can all contribute to the amount of stress a person experiences. For instance, individuals with lower socioeconomic status might face constant financial pressures, limited access to healthcare, and less social support, all of which can significantly increase their stress levels.

Moreover, these theories emphasise the importance of social roles and expectations. For example, someone who is a primary caregiver might experience stress not only from their caregiving duties but also from perceived societal expectations and pressures to perform the role in an ideal or perfect way. Stress is compounded when a person feels that they fail to meet these expectations or lack adequate support. These factors are known as the exposure hypothesis and the vulnerability hypothesis, with exposure to stressors being the likelihood of stressors occurring based on social factors, while vulnerability relates to how the individual reacts to any given stressors (Surachman and Almeida, 2018). Social Stress Theories also highlight the role of social support networks, as explained by Pearlin et al. (1981). Strong, supportive relationships can act as a buffer against stress, providing emotional support, practical help, and a sense of belonging. Conversely, social isolation or negative social interactions can exacerbate stress, increasing feelings of loneliness and helplessness.

Psychological Understandings of Stress

On a psychological level, stress involves a range of cognitive and emotional responses. The way in which we perceive and interpret stressors through cognitive appraisal determines our emotional reactions and coping strategies (Yeo and Ong, 2024). Psychological theories, such as the Transactional

Model of Stress and Coping (Lazarus, 1966; Lazarus and Folkman, 1984), highlight the importance of individual differences in stress perception and management. Effective coping mechanisms, such as problem-solving and emotional regulation, can mitigate the negative effects of stress, while mal-adaptive coping strategies may worsen stress and its consequences (Polizzi and Lynn, 2021).

Transactional Model of Stress and Coping

The Transactional Model (Lazarus, 1966; Lazarus and Folkman, 1984) emphasises that stress is not just about the external events we face, but also about how we perceive and respond to these events. It views stress as a transaction between the individual and their environment, highlighting the role of cognitive appraisal and coping strategies. There are three stages to this processing: primary appraisal, secondary appraisal, and coping strategies.

1. **Primary Appraisal**: This is the first step in the stress response process. When faced with a potential stressor, we assess its significance, asking ourselves questions like: "Is this situation harmful, threatening, or chal-lenging?" This primary appraisal helps us determine whether we should feel stressed and how severe the situation is.

2. **Secondary Appraisal**: After evaluating the stressor, we then assess our ability to cope with it. We consider the resources and options available to us, asking questions like "Can I handle this?" and "What can I do to manage this situation?" This step is crucial because it influences our emotional response and the coping strategies we choose.

3. **Coping Strategies**: Based on our appraisals, we select coping strategies to manage the stressor. These strategies can be problem-focused, where we take action to change the situation, or emotion-focused, where we try to manage our emotional response. For example, if an individual is stressed about a work deadline, a problem-focused approach might involve cre-ating a detailed plan to complete the task, while an emotion-focused approach might involve talking to a friend to express feelings and gain emotional support.

The Transactional Model highlights that stress is a subjective experience, shaped by our thoughts, perceptions, and coping abilities. It underscores the importance of cognitive processes in determining how we experience stress and the effectiveness of our coping mechanisms. Understanding this model empowers us to recognise the pivotal role of our mindset in stress management. By improving our cognitive appraisal skills and developing effective coping strategies, we can better navigate the challenges that life throws our way. As healthcare professionals, it also enables us to understand the reasons behind individual differences in resilience and coping.

Understanding the Life Course Perspective

The Life Course Perspective (Pearlin et al., 2005) emphasises that experiences, including stress, are shaped by the timing and sequence of life events. It looks at how key transitions and social roles influence our stress levels and coping mechanisms over time, exploring trajectory, transitions, and timing, alongside the cultural context, as described in more detail in Box 3.1.

Box 3.1 Influences on Responses to Stress across the Life Course

Firstly, trajectory, the long-term patterns of stability and change in a person's life, can influence stress and coping strategies. For instance, an individual's career trajectory might include various roles, promotions, and periods of unemployment. It may be changes in trajectory that have impacted Alice's ability to cope.

Secondly, transitions and significant life changes, such as graduating from university, getting married, or retiring, can be sources of stress, but they also present opportunities for growth and adaptation. How we navigate these transitions is crucial to our overall wellbeing. The Transactional Model (Lazarus, 1966; Lazarus and Folkman, 1984) might provide clues as to whether each transition is perceived positively or negatively.

Thirdly, the timing of life events matters. Experiencing a major transition like parenthood or job loss earlier or later than expected can affect how we perceive and cope with the associated stress. For example, becoming a parent as a teenager may pose different stressors compared to becoming a parent in our thirties. This could relate to the social elements of stress already explored (Surachman and Almeida, 2018) and is explained in the Life Course Perspective in terms of how our lives are linked to other people's. These social connections influence our stress experiences. For instance, caring for an ageing parent can be both a source of stress and a tremendously meaningful experience.

Finally, the wider contexts of our cultural background and the social norms by which we live, shape our stress experiences. Cultural expectations about career success, family roles, and ageing can influence how we perceive and cope with stress at specific times of life.

The Life Course Perspective highlights that stress is not a static experience; it evolves as we move through different stages of life. By considering the timing of events, the interconnectedness of our lives, and the broader cultural context, this perspective provides a holistic understanding of stress. It reminds us that our stress experiences are not isolated incidents but part of a larger narrative that unfolds over time. The parts played by social experiences and psychological coping mechanisms highlight why having a holistic understanding and carrying out thorough assessments are an essential prerequisite for delivering person-centred care.

Understanding the Bio-Psycho-Social Signs and Symptoms of Stress

Stress manifests in various ways, affecting biological, psychological, and social wellbeing in an interactional way. When one of these systems is impacted, this can spread to, or influence, our perceptions of other aspects of life. Recognising these signs and symptoms can help us manage stress more effectively as well as help in the process of seeking appropriate support. These are identified in Table 3.2 below.

Absence of the signs or symptoms identified in Table 3.2 indicates that the body is operating at baseline and is in a state of normal functioning, meaning that the body and mind are at rest, free from the immediate effects of stress. Chronic stress can make it challenging to return to this baseline

Table 3.2 Biological, Social and Psychological Signs of Stress

Social	• Social withdrawal • Relationship strain • Decreased social functioning (work/education)
Biological	• Increased heart rate • Muscle tension • Digestive issues • Headaches • Sleep disturbance • Fatigue
Psychological	• Anxiety • Depression • Irritability • Difficulty concentrating • Emotional exhaustion/burnout

due to depleted resources, dysregulations of the HPA axis, or the presence of habitual response patterns.

Resources are likely to become depleted where the body's constant state of alertness reduces reserves of physical and emotional resources, making recovery more difficult. Similarly, prolonged stress can lead to dysregulation of the HPA axis, impairing the body's ability to shut off the stress response. Lastly, repeated stress can condition the body to remain in a heightened state of alertness, making relaxation and recovery harder to achieve and resulting in a habitual stress response.

Assessing Risk

Risk factors for distress, stress, anger, and agitation are dynamic and context-dependent, influenced by individual experiences, environmental triggers, and fluctuating psychological states. Traditional risk assessments in clinical practice often rely on static models that attempt to predict future behaviour based on historical data. However, these assessments may lack precision, as they struggle to account for the fluid nature of risk, particularly in mental health settings. A study by Nathan and Bhandari (2024) highlights that risk assessments often fail to provide usable probability estimates for individual cases, leading to over-reliance on categorical judgements rather than nuanced, person-centred evaluations. Additionally, the Care Quality Commission (2024) emphasises the importance of holistic, person-centred risk management, cautioning against rigid assessment frameworks that may overlook real-time changes in distress levels. NHS England (2024) further underscores the need for adaptive risk assessment models, particularly in integrated care systems where multiple factors – such as wider socioeconomic conditions and access to support – can rapidly shift an individual's risk profile. These findings suggest that clinicians should prioritise continuous monitoring and flexible intervention strategies rather than relying solely on static risk assessment tools.

Despite this, assessment and planning of patient care are a core part of the healthcare professional's role (Ajibade, 2021). While the use of risk assessment tools is cautioned, professionals should follow a structured approach to assess the risk of aggressive behaviour or expressions of distress and frustration by patients. Here's a step-by-step guide:

1. Identify Potential Triggers

    Understand the factors that might provoke agitation, such as long waiting times, lack of information, or personal history of violence. Recognising these triggers helps in anticipating and preventing incidents of concern.

    If a therapeutic relationship has not first been established, individuals may not be able or willing to identify what triggers their agitation and anger, when asked. In this case, while care should always be person-centred and tailored to the person in front of you, taking into consideration some common triggers can help. These might include triggers from their current situation, like feeling that they are not being listened to or not agreeing with their care plan (particularly when held under the Mental Health Act (1983)). Alternatively, there may be triggers from previous experiences such as someone with a history of sexual abuse struggling with being touched.

2. Conduct a Risk Assessment

    Perform a comprehensive risk assessment that evaluates the likelihood and potential impact of aggressive behaviour. This involves:

    a. Evaluating the patient's mental, emotional, and physical condition.

    b. Considering the effects of medical conditions, medications, or substance use.*

    c. Reviewing the patient's history of challenging or aggressive behaviour.

It is important to remember that risk is fluid; any risk assessments should be combined with clinical judgement, and structured risk tools should not be relied upon in isolation (Nathan and Bhandari, 2024).

3. Implement Control Measures

   Based on the risk assessment, implement appropriate control measures to minimise the risk associated with expressions of anger. These measures might include:

   a. Environmental modifications, such as ensuring a safe and calm environment.

   b. Staff training on de-escalation techniques and effective communication.

   c. Clear instructions and protocols for responding to actions that cause concern.

   While implementing control measures, it is also important to avoid being risk-averse, taking positive risks where they are likely to be of therapeutic benefit to the patient, and avoid blanket restrictions. The Mental Health Act (1983) states blanket restrictions (such as removing all charging leads in inpatient settings due to risk of ligaturing) should be avoided unless they are justified as necessary and proportionate to the presenting risks, and this should be regularly reviewed.

4. Monitor and Review

   Regularly monitor the effectiveness of the control measures and review the risk assessment. This helps in identifying any changes in the patient's condition or behaviour, to adjust the approach accordingly.

5. Involve the Patient

   Engage the patient in the risk assessment process, where possible. This can help in understanding their perspective and building a collaborative approach to managing their expressions of anger and distress.

6. Document and Communicate

   Document all risk assessments, control measures, and incidents of concern. Ensure that all staff members are aware of any potential risks and the strategies in place to manage them.

By following these steps, professionals can effectively assess and manage the risk of expressions of extreme distress, ensuring the safety and wellbeing of both patients and staff.

Tools for Now: Small Changes That Can Make a Big Difference

The effective management of anger and distress involves various strategies and tools that are designed to help individuals regain control and respond constructively. They include:

- Cognitive behavioural techniques are widely used to address the root causes of anger, such as identifying and challenging negative thoughts.
- Relaxation methods, including deep breathing exercises and progressive muscle relaxation, can help reduce physiological arousal.
- Mindfulness practices encourage present-moment awareness and emotional regulation.
- Communication skills training to enhance assertiveness and reduce conflicts.
- Professional support, such as therapy or counselling, offering personalised guidance and strategies tailored to individual needs.

Together, these tools empower individuals to manage anger and distress in healthy ways.

Coaching someone to identify and challenge their negative thoughts involves guiding them through a process of self-awareness and cognitive restructuring (Purdon, 2021). Here is a step-by-step approach on how healthcare professionals can coach someone to develop these skills:

Step 1: Awareness

This involves paying attention to internal dialogue, which can be supported by keeping a thought diary, noting down the content of thoughts, and any emotional response to these. Ultimately, this can help with recognising patterns and triggers.

Step 2: Identifying Cognitive Distortions

It is essential to support the individual to understand common cognitive distortions. These are irrational thought patterns that often lead to negative thinking. Examples include:

1. All-or-nothing thinking: viewing situations in black and white terms.

2. Over-generalisation: making broad statements based on limited evidence.

3. Catastrophising: expecting the worst possible outcome.

4. Personalisation: blaming oneself for events outside one's control.

It is most helpful if the person can be taught to recognise these kinds of distortions in their own thinking.

Step 3: Challenging Negative Thoughts

Once a negative thought has been identified, coach the person in ways to challenge its validity. They can be encouraged to ask questions around the themes of evidence, alternatives, realism, and impact, as demonstrated in Table 3.3.

Table 3.3 Approaches to Questioning Negative Thoughts

Types of questions	Examples:
Evidence	What evidence supports this thought? What evidence contradicts it?
Alternatives	Are there alternative explanations or perspectives?
Realism	Is this thought realistic? Is it based on facts or assumptions?
Impact	How does thinking this way make them feel? How would they feel if they thought differently?

Encouraging the person to write down their responses to these questions can help in breaking down and examining negative thoughts in logical and systematic ways that can be repeated by the individual independently, once they are familiar with the process.

Step 4: Reframing

Guide the person to reframe the negative thought into a more balanced and realistic one. For example, if they think: "I'm terrible at my job", help them reframe it to: "I had a challenging day, but I've succeeded in the past, and I can improve with practice."

Step 5: Practice and Reinforcement

Encourage regular practice of these steps. Consistent application helps to embed new, healthier thought patterns. You can also reinforce their progress and celebrate small victories, which builds confidence and motivation.

Thinking about Language

Using terms like "aggression" or "aggressive" to describe a patient or service user can be problematic and detrimental to their longer-term wellbeing for a variety of reasons. These are explored below.

Stigmatisation

The words that we use can lead to bias and stigma in the delivery of health and social care (Valdez, 2021). Labelling someone as aggressive can lead others to view the person as dangerous or difficult, before they have got to know them, which can contribute to social isolation and discrimination. This can be particularly harmful for individuals already struggling with mental health issues, as it can exacerbate feelings of shame and alienation.

Misunderstanding

Aggressive actions and verbalisations can often be a symptom of underlying issues such as anxiety, trauma, or frustration, or an unmet need (Valimaki et al., 2022), as well as agitation and irritability being a side effect of some medications used in mental health. By focusing solely on the behaviour and labelling it as aggression, professionals might overlook the root causes. This can prevent the person from receiving the appropriate support, care, and intervention they need to address underlying problems.

Escalation

Using terms like "aggressive" can create a self-fulfilling prophecy (Jussim, 2012). If a person is repeatedly labelled as aggressive, they might start to internalise this label and act accordingly. This can lead to a cycle of behaviour, where the person repeatedly feels misunderstood and reacts with more intense emotions.

Communication Breakdown

Describing someone as aggressive can hinder effective communication (Sharkiya, 2023). It can create an adversarial relationship between the professional and the patient, making it harder to build trust and rapport. This can impede the therapeutic process and make it more challenging to work together towards positive outcomes.

Bias and Prejudice

Professionals might unconsciously apply the label of aggression more readily to certain groups of people due to biases based on race, gender, homelessness, or socioeconomic status (Valdez, 2021). This can lead to unequal treatment and reinforce systemic inequalities in healthcare.

Alternative Approaches

Instead of labelling behaviour as aggressive, professionals can use more specific and non-judgemental language (Linehan, 1993). For example, they can describe specific actions such as "tense muscles" or "loud voice" or describe what appear to be the underlying emotions, such as "frustration" or "distress." This approach focuses on understanding the person's experience and finding constructive ways to address their needs.

Validation and Communication: The Importance of Listening

Effective management of distress and stress, especially in healthcare and therapeutic settings, relies heavily on validation and communication, as well as the use of active listening skills. Each of these elements is essential for building trust, understanding, and for providing appropriate support.

Validation

Validation involves acknowledging and accepting a person's feelings and experiences without judgement (Fruzzetti and Ruork, 2019). For individuals experiencing stress or distress, validation can be incredibly powerful. It communicates that their emotions are real, relevant, and understandable, which can reduce feelings of isolation and frustration. By validating a person's feelings, professionals can help de-escalate strong feelings and create a safe space for open communication. This approach fosters trust and encourages individuals to express their emotions more constructively.

Communication

Clear and compassionate communication is essential in managing distress and stress (Sharkiya, 2023). Professionals must convey information in a way that is easy to understand and free from jargon. Effective communication includes not only speaking but also non-verbal cues, such as body language and facial expressions, which can convey empathy and understanding. By maintaining open lines of communication, professionals can help individuals feel more comfortable to share their thoughts and feelings. This openness can prevent misunderstandings and reduce the likelihood of expressions of distress, such as agitation and anger.

Listening Skills

Active listening is a fundamental skill in managing distress and stress. It goes beyond simply hearing words and involves fully engaging with the speaker, understanding their perspective, and responding thoughtfully. Active listening helps in identifying the underlying causes of a person's distress and can help in gathering crucial information to inform their approach to addressing the person's needs and concerns. This can lead to more effective interventions and support. It also demonstrates empathy and respect by supporting the individual to know that they are heard and valued.

Together, validation, communication, and active listening form the cornerstone of effective management of stress and distress. They enable professionals to build rapport, understand the individual's needs, and provide tailored support that addresses the root causes of distress. By creating a supportive environment, practitioners can help individuals navigate their emotions and reduce the impact of stress and distress on their wellbeing.

De-escalation Techniques

When encountering a person who is becoming stressed, frustrated, or overtly agitated and angry, quick use of de-escalation techniques can support the management of the situation. Outwardly maintaining a calm demeanour is crucial, as *your* calmness can help diffuse tension and reassure the individual in distress, as well as using mirroring techniques to reduce their levels of agitation, anger and distress. This is supported by adopting an open and non-threatening posture, which in itself supports de-escalation, as the information then given subconsciously via non-verbal communication, promotes a feeling of safety rather than threat. Try to avoid crossed arms, standing too close, or making sudden movements, all of which may be perceived as acts of challenge or aggression by the person who is distressed. Instead, use open gestures while maintaining a safe distance.

As not feeling listened to can be a trigger for the escalation of feelings, it is helpful to give each person options and involve them in decision-making. This can help them feel more in control and reduce feelings of helplessness. While being empathic, it is also important to set clear boundaries and not to allow abusive actions or speech in healthcare environments. Let the person know what behaviours are acceptable and what are not, in a respectful and non-confrontational manner. Finally, if the situation escalates, do not hesitate to call for additional support from colleagues or security personnel. It's important to ensure the safety of everyone involved.

Reducing and Managing Stress and Distress: Specialist Approaches

Anger Management Programmes

In the UK, specialist services for anger management offer a range of interventions designed to help individuals understand and manage their anger more effectively (Toohey, 2021). These usually consist of individual or group therapy or support options, and involve supporting the person to set their goals, engage in an intervention, and then prevent relapse into previous behaviours. These might be completed in an anger management programme (Illman and Brown, 2016), or as part of another intervention, depending on clinician skills and training. Anger management programmes typically involve group or individual sessions where participants learn techniques to control their anger, including relaxation exercises, communication skills training, and strategies for coping with stress and frustration.

Cognitive Behavioural Therapy (CBT) is a commonly used approach in anger management programmes, which helps individuals identify and challenge negative thought patterns contributing to anger, while also developing healthier ways of thinking and responding (Nakao et al., 2021). Mindfulness practices and relaxation techniques, such as deep breathing, meditation, and progressive muscle relaxation, can help individuals stay calm and reduce the physiological arousal associated with anger (Toohey, 2021). It might be appropriate to signpost self-help resources, such as books, online courses, and apps, which individuals can use to practice anger management techniques at their own pace, such as the online workbook provided by NHS Inform (2025).

Trauma- and Violence-Informed Care

Trauma- and violence-informed care is crucial when working with distressed or agitated patients because it acknowledges the profound impact that trauma can have on an individual's mental, physical, and emotional wellbeing (Office for Health Improvement and Disparities, 2022). This means practitioners recognise that aggressive or distressed behaviour may be a result of past trauma or ongoing stress. By recognising these underlying causes, professionals can address the root issues rather than just the symptoms.

A trauma-informed approach considers how professionals can create a safe and supportive environment for patients. This involves setting clear boundaries, ensuring physical and emotional safety, and fostering a sense of trust and security, as well as being mindful of triggers and avoiding actions or words that could cause the patient to relive their trauma, which would be retraumatising (Office for Health Improvement and Disparities, 2022).

Professionals should give patients a voice in their care, respecting their choices, and working together to develop coping strategies and solutions. This is done by placing emphasis on the importance of the therapeutic relationship and building trust and rapport. This trust is essential for effective communication and for encouraging patients to engage in their treatment and recovery. Ultimately, trauma-informed care can lead to better health outcomes. By addressing the holistic needs of the patient and providing compassionate care, professionals can help patients heal and manage their stress and distress more effectively. Incorporating trauma- and violence-informed care into healthcare practices ensures that patients receive the understanding, support, and respect they need to navigate their challenges and work towards recovery.

Summary of Learning Points

This chapter has explored the following theoretical and practical approaches to understanding stress and distress:

- A review of biological understandings of stress explored the SAM and HPA axis pathways, identifying how they work together to make up physiological responses to short-term and prolonged stress.
- In addition, social understandings of stress, including Social Stress Theory, as well as psychological understandings of stress, such as the Transactional Model of Stress and Coping, are considered alongside each other, contributing to our understanding of stress as being influenced by and expressed through bio-psycho-social factors and symptoms.
- A consideration of the Life Course Perspective adds a further aspect to the multifactorial dimensions of stress, including how key periods and transitions within the lifespan can influence experiences of stress.
- Evidence-based tools for supporting people, including risk assessment and communication approaches, have been presented.
- A discussion of the specialist interventions available for anger management and the importance of taking a trauma-informed approach to the prevention and management of stress and distress is outlined.

Questions for Reflection and Discussion

1. How can you work in ways that help to ensure that you understand the underlying causes of a patient's stress and distress?
2. What steps can you take to create a safe and supportive environment for patients, including taking a trauma-informed approach and validating the feelings of patients and service users?

3. What steps could you take in your communication to increase clarity, compassion, and the use of active listening skills, as well as empathic responses?

4. How thorough is your process for identifying potential triggers for distress and stress, to ensure that you avoid retraumatising patients and service users? How could you further involve patients and service users in the risk assessment process to better understand their needs?

5. How can you integrate approaches to supporting patients and service users to have greater awareness of their own thinking and how they can challenge their negative thoughts?

Recommended Follow-up Reading

Albeti, R. and Knaus, W.J. (2021). *The Cognitive Behavioral Workbook for Anger: A Step-by-Step Program for Success*. Oakland, CA: Impact Publishing/New Harbinger Publications.

Centre for Clinical Interventions (2019). Looking after yourself: Tolerating distress. Available online at: https://www.cci.health.wa.gov.au/Resources/Looking-After-Yourself/Tolerating-Distress. [Accessed 20th August 2025].

Housden, S. (2025). (ed) *Trauma Informed Practice for Nurses and Allied Health Professionals*. Abingdon: Routledge.

Nathan, R. and Bhandari, S. (2024). Risk assessment in clinical practice: A framework for decision-making in real-world complex systems. *BJPsych Advances*. 30(1): 53–63.

NHS Inform (2025). Problems with anger self-help guide. Available online at: https://www.nhsinform.scot/illnesses-and-conditions/mental-health/mental-health-self-help-guides/problems-with-anger-self-help-guide/. [Accessed 10th February 2025].

References

Ajibade, B. (2021). Assessing the patient's needs and planning effective care. *British Journal of Nursing*. 30(20): 1166–1171.

Care Quality Commission (2024). Assessment framework. Available online at: https://www.cqc.org.uk/guidance-regulation/providers/assessment/single-assessment-framework/safe/involving-people-manage-risk. [Accessed 24th April 2025].

Cohen, S. and Willis, T.A. (1985). Stress, social support, and the buffering hypothesis. *Psychological Bulletin*. 98(2): 310–357.

Fruzzetti, A.E. and Ruork, A.K. (2019). Validation principles and practices in dialectical behavioural therapy. In M.A. Swales (Ed.), *The Oxford Handbook of Dialectical Behaviour Therapy*. Oxford: Oxford University Press, pp. 325–344.

Illman, N.A. and Brown, J.S.L. (2016). Reaching out to problem anger: Assessing the effectiveness of one-day cognitive behavioural workshops in a community setting in the UK. *Behavioural and Cognitive Psychotherapy*. 44(5): 615–619.

Jussim, L. (2012). *Social Perception and Social Reality: Why Accuracy Dominates Bias and Self-Fulfilling Prophecy*. Oxford: Oxford Academic: Online edition.

Lazarus, R.S. (1966). *Psychological Stress and the Coping Process*. New York and Maidenhead: McGraw Hill.

Lazarus, R.S. and Folkman, S. (1984). *Stress, Appraisal, and Coping*. New York: Springer Publishing.

Linehan, M.M. (1993). *Cognitive Behavioural Therapy for Borderline Personality Disorder*. New York: Guildford Press.

McCarty, R. (2016). *The fight-or-flight response: A cornerstone of stress research*. In G. Fink (Ed.), *Stress: Concepts, Cognition, Emotion, and Behaviour*. Cambridge, MA: Academic Press, pp. 33–37.

Mental Health Act (1983). Available online at: https://www.legislation.gov.uk/ukpga/1983/20/contents. [Accessed 10th February 2025].

Nakao, M., Shirotsuki, K. and Sugaya, N. (2021). Cognitive-behavioral therapy for management of mental health and stress-related disorders: Recent advances in technique and technologies. *BioPsychoSocial Medicine*. 15(16): 1–4.

Nathan, R. and Bhandari, S. (2024). Risk assessment in clinical practice: A framework for decision-making in real-world complex systems. *BJPsych Advances*. 30(1): 53–63.

NHS England (2024). Principles for assessing and managing risks across integrated care systems. Available online at: https://www.england.nhs.uk/long-read/principles-for-assessing-and-managing-risks-across-integrated-care-systems/. [Accessed 10th February 2025].

NHS Inform (2025). Problems with anger self-help guide. Available online at: https://www.nhsinform.scot/illnesses-and-conditions/mental-health/mental-health-self-help-guides/problems-with-anger-self-help-guide/. [Accessed 10th February 2025].

Office for Health Improvement and Disparities (2022). Working definition of trauma-informed practice. Available online at: https://www.gov.uk/government/publications/working-definition-of-trauma-informed-practice/working-definition-of-trauma-informed-practice. [Accessed 10th February 2025].

Pearlin, L.I., Menaghan, E.G., Liberman, M.A. and Mullen, J.T. (1981). The stress process. *Journal of Health and Social Behavior*. 22(4): 337–356.

Pearlin, L.I., Schieman, S., Faxio, E.M. and Meersman, S.C. (2005). Stress, health, and the life course: Some conceptual perspectives. *Journal of Health and Social Behaviour*. 46(2): 205–219.

Polizzi, C.P. and Lynn, S.J. (2021). Regulating emotionality to manage adversity: A systematic review of the relation between emotion regulation and psychological resilience. *Cognitive Therapy and Research*. 45: 577–597.

Purdon, C. (2021). Cognitive restructuring. In A. Wenzel (Ed.), *Handbook of Cognitive Behavioural Therapy: Overview and Approaches*. Washington, DC: American Psychological Association, pp. 207–234.

Ravi, M., Miller, A.H. and Michopoulos, V. (2021). The immunology of stress and the impact of inflammation on the brain and behaviour. *BJPsych Advances*. 27(3): 158–165.

Sarmiento, L.F., Rios-Florez, J.A., Rincon Uribe, F.A., Lima, R.R., Kalenscher, T., Gouveia Jr, A. and Nitsch, F.J. (2024). Do stress hormones influence choice? A systematic review of pharmacological interventions on the HPA axis and/or SAM system. *Social Cognitive and Affective Neuroscience*. 19(1): 1–17.

Sharkiya, S.H. (2023). Quality communication can improve patient-centred health outcomes among older patients: A rapid review. *BMC Health Services Research*. 23: 1–14.

Surachman, A. and Almeida, D.M. (2018). Stress and coping theory across the adult lifespan. *Oxford Research Encyclopedia of Psychology*. Available online at: https://doi.org/10.1093/acrefore/9780190236557.013.341. [Accessed 11th August 2025].

Toohey, M.J. (2021). Cognitive behavioral therapy for anger management. In A Wenzel (Ed.), *Handbook of Cognitive Behavioral Therapy: Applications*. Washington, DC: American Psychological Association, pp. 331–359.

Valdez, A. (2021). Words matter: Labelling, bias and stigma in nursing. *Journal of Advanced Nursing*. 77(11): 4291–4598.

Valimaki, M., Lantta, T., Lam, Y.T.J., Cheung, T., Cheng, P.Y.I., Ip, G. and Bressington, D. (2022). Perceptions of patient aggression in psychiatric hospitals: A qualitative study using focus groups with nurses, patients, and informal caregivers. *BMC Psychiatry*. 22: 1–14.

Yeo, G.C. and Ong, D.C. (2024). Associations between cognitive appraisals and emotions: A meta-analytic review. *Psychological Bulletin*. 150(12): 1140–1471.

Understanding Non-Suicidal Self-Harm

4

Louise Cherrill and
Hannah Bailey

Case Study

Sophie's Story

I first started self-harming when I was in high school. I am not sure if I was the first one in my friendship group and two others then followed, or they just shared with me they were doing it too after they found out I was. It was a way to help me cope with how I was feeling – depressed – due to relentless bullying from 'popular girls'. I did it when I felt as though I was going to explode, like a bottle of coke dropped down the stairs. It took the lid off in a controlled way. Sometimes I would do it to punish myself, when I felt like I deserved it. Sometimes it was just to feel something, because I felt nothing but darkness and sadness.

I remember the first time a medical professional saw it, and they said: "Oh it's just superficial", which left me feeling like it wasn't good enough for them to care about or for them to help me. Perhaps I had to try harder to be taken seriously, because their dismissal of my self-harm as superficial, in some way also dismissed my pain as superficial.

I self-harmed on and off into my 20s, but then I stopped. It never went away though. Much like I have friends who have quit smoking and who say that they really want a cigarette when they have a bad day, my mind still travels back to cutting myself to manage stress and difficult times. However, unlike my friends who can share how they are going to have a bottle of wine, a large pizza, go for a run, smoke,

---

DOI: 10.4324/9781003635611-5

or whatever coping strategies they employ to manage their feelings, I cannot share the feelings I have about wanting to self-harm, without feeling judged and experiencing shame. The pressure of hiding these thoughts to avoid other people's responses and to avoid shame and judgement, can be so lonely and isolating. People just don't understand self-harm.

Introduction

Self-harm is a complex and multifaceted issue that has garnered significant attention in both medical and psychological fields. According to the National Institute for Health and Care Excellence (NICE), self-harm refers to any act of self-injury or self-poisoning carried out by an individual, irrespective of their intention to die (NICE, 2022). On the other hand, researcher Matthew Nock defines Non-Suicidal Self-Injury (NSSI) as self-inflicted damage to body tissue without suicidal intent and for purposes that are not socially sanctioned (Nock, 2012). The distinction between self-harm and NSSI lies primarily in the presence or absence of suicidal intent, with NSSI explicitly excluding behaviours which have suicidal intent.

Behaviours constituting self-harm include cutting, burning, or hitting oneself, among others (Wood, 2009). However, other behaviours such as eating disorders and alcohol or substance misuse are sometimes viewed as forms of self-harm due to their self-destructive nature and potential to cause bodily harm (Wood, 2009). Understanding the nuances and definitions of these terms is crucial for developing effective interventions and support systems for those affected by self-harm, but also for ensuring that the care provided is meaningful and patient-centred (Hetrick et al., 2020).

Interpreting self-harm statistics is challenging due to the secretive nature of these behaviours, with many incidents never coming to the attention of professionals. Additionally, variations in how professionals classify self-harm, along with delays in the publication of statistics, further complicate the accuracy of these figures. In the UK, the Adult Psychiatric Morbidity Survey suggests approximately 1 in 14 people self-harm during their lifetime (McManus et al., 2016). Globally, the World Health Organization (WHO, 2019) reports that self-harm is a significant public health concern, with millions of cases occurring annually.

Chapter Aims

This chapter focuses on providing a comprehensive overview of trauma and includes information and discussion around ideas which explore:

- The functions of self-harm as a behaviour.
- Understandings of contagion.
- Ways of helping patients and service users to manage urges to self-harm.
- Specialist interventions for managing self-harm.

Reasons behind Self-Harm

Self-harm has long been misunderstood as a method of attention-seeking or a cry for help. These ideas perpetuate the shame, stigma, and secrecy experienced by individuals (Sadath et al., 2024) such as Sophie in this chapter's case study. In 2007, Klonsky conducted a comprehensive literature review to understand the functions of self-harm, identifying 18 empirical studies on the topic. This review collated evidence to explain the various functions of self-injury. As seen in Sophie's case, the reasons for self-harm may change over time, and the different models and explanations can overlap or occur concurrently (Klonsky, 2007). Klonsky's review remains relevant to contemporary practice, as researchers have continued to use these models and have consistently found similar reasons for self-harm in their studies over the past 20 years.

The most common function of self-harm identified in research literature is regulation of affect (mood), where self-harm is used to reduce or remove negative feelings (Klonsky, 2007). Self-harm can thereby become a maladaptive strategy for emotional regulation, which helps individuals manage intense negative emotions. Research indicates that self-harm behaviours, such as cutting or burning, can temporarily relieve emotional distress by releasing endorphins and providing a distraction from emotional pain (Wolff et al., 2019). The use of this type of coping mechanism can be particularly prevalent among people who struggle to manage their emotions in more constructive and healthier ways. Some studies have shown a significant association between emotional dysregulation and self-harming actions

(Rogier et al., 2020; Hitchens et al., 2019). This highlights the importance of addressing underlying emotional issues in treatment.

The role of emotional dysregulation in self-harming has also been explored by Linehan (1993). She explains that individuals can have an innate sensitivity to emotions in a similar way to which some people may be sensitive to laundry detergent or lactose. Such individuals are more likely to experience emotional dysregulation if they also grew up in invalidating environments, as described in the biosocial model (Linehan, 1993). Emotional dysregulation refers to the inability to manage or respond to emotional experiences in a controlled and appropriate manner (D'Agostino et al., 2017). This often involves intense and prolonged emotional reactions, difficulty in soothing oneself, and challenges in returning to a baseline emotional state. Where alternative coping skills have not been acquired, self-harm can become a way of regulating emotions.

Research has identified both psychological (Suyemoto, 1998; Brown et al., 2002) and biological (Weinberg and Klonsky, 2012) pathways that explain the reduction in negative arousal that occurs upon self-harming. Self-injury can provide sensations and elicit physiological arousal, contributing to its effectiveness as a coping mechanism (Nixon et al., 2002). This function of self-harm was supported by a study where 12% of the sample (103 adolescents, 75 of whom were female) reported engaging in self-harm. Of these participants, 79% identified "getting relief from a terrible state of mind", and 43% cited emotional regulation as one of their motivations (Doyle et al., 2017: 138).

Self-harm can become a deeply ingrained coping strategy due to the immediate relief it provides from emotional distress. This relief is linked to the release of endorphins and other chemicals in the brain, which temporarily numb emotional pain. Over time, individuals may come to rely on self-harm as a primary method of coping, leading to an addictive pattern of behaviour (Blasco-Frontecilla et al., 2016). The addictive nature of self-harm is supported by research that shows how the brain's reward system is activated during self-injury, in a similar way to how it responds to addictive substances (Wang et al., 2025). This activation creates a positive feedback loop, where the temporary relief reinforces the behaviour, making it increasingly difficult to break the cycle. Studies have found that the urge to self-harm can become compulsive, with individuals feeling a strong desire to enact these thoughts, even when they recognise that it has harmful consequences (Himelein-Wachowiak et al., 2022).

Self-harm can serve as a mechanism to feel something or to counter-act dissociation for people who otherwise describe feeling numb (Klonsky, 2007). This was cited by 8% of participants in the study by Doyle et al. (2017). Additionally, as described by Sophie in our case study, and reported by 38% of the adolescents in Doyle's study (Doyle et al., 2017), self-harm can function as a method of self-punishment (Klonsky, 2007). Self-harm may also serve to influence others, such as demonstrating the level of distress being experienced, to another person (Klonsky, 2007). However, only 11% of the adolescents in Doyle's study indicated this as their reason (Doyle et al., 2017). The misconception of self-harm as "just attention-seeking" continues to feed the secrecy and perceived shame surrounding such actions.

It is uncomfortable, difficult, and controversial to consider that there might be positive aspects to someone engaging in self-harming behaviours, but evidence suggests it can be protective against suicide. For example, self-harm can serve to avoid acting on suicidal urges (Suyemoto, 1998) or to prevent suicidal ideation (Himber, 1994). When self-harm is used as a coping strategy, preventing it can inadvertently increase the risk of suicide attempts (Klonsky, 2007; Edwards and Hewitt, 2011). Consider your own coping strategies, such as consuming food or wine, or participating in exercise, and imagine the impact on your mental state if you were suddenly prevented from engaging in these activities. For most people, this would result in increased stress and anxiety.

However, any understanding of the potentially protective functions of self-harm must be balanced with the known risk of self-injurious actions being associated with an increased risk of suicide (Chan et al., 2018). Thus, both preventing and allowing self-harm can carry potential risks of suicide (Edwards and Hewitt, 2011). This dilemma is particularly relevant for service users admitted to acute inpatient services. The ethical considerations of this issue are thoughtfully discussed in Edwards and Hewitt (2011).

In practice, managing risks around self-harm involves balancing harm minimisation or safer self-harm approaches (NICE, 2022). These methods may not be suitable for every patient and should always be applied in line with local policies, professional guidance, multidisciplinary team working, and NICE guidelines (2022). When appropriate, harm minimisation strategies might include teaching distraction techniques to prevent acting on urges, encouraging self-care of wounds (when medically appropriate), and supporting the reduction of scarring (NICE, 2022). It can also involve ensuring that implements used for harm are clean and that wounds are kept clean to reduce the risk of infection (NICE, 2022). Importantly, these approaches should always work towards replacing self-harm with more adaptive coping strategies (NICE, 2022).

Understanding Social Contagion

Social contagion theory states that behaviours, emotions, and psychological phenomena can spread spontaneously within social groups through imitation and modelling (Riggio and Riggio, 2023). This theory suggests that individuals are influenced by the actions and emotions of those around them, leading to the rapid dissemination of behaviours and ideas. Social contagion can occur in various contexts, including health-related behaviours, emotional states, and even psychological symptoms. For example, research has shown that behaviours such as smoking, obesity, and happiness can spread through social networks, as individuals tend to mirror the behaviours of their peers (Christakis and Fowler, 2013). This phenomenon is particularly relevant in understanding the spread of self-harm behaviours among adolescents, where exposure to self-harm within social groups or through media can lead to an increase in similar behaviours (Wester et al., 2018).

Evidence has shown that having a family member or friend who self-harms is statistically the most significant predictor of self-harming behaviours (O'Connor et al., 2012). Having a friend who self-harms can increase the risk of engaging in similar actions by a factor of three (You et al., 2013). This phenomenon, known as the contagion effect, refers to the spread of self-harm behaviours through social groups, in a similar way to how a virus spreads. Contagion often involves self-harm by an adolescent, which takes place after discussing self-harm or after being exposed to it in the media (Berger et al., 2014).

Having a best friend who self-harms is a strong predictor of self-harming behaviour, while belonging to a peer group of adolescents who self-harm can increase the frequency of these actions (You et al., 2013). This is concerning, as adolescents tend to gravitate towards and befriend those experiencing similar problems, a phenomenon known as the selection effect (Doyle et al., 2015). According to social learning theory (Bandura, 1977), individuals may then model this behaviour. A qualitative study by O'Connor et al. (2012) examined differences between adolescents who think about self-harm (ideators) and those who engage in self-harming behaviours (enactors) with a sample of 5,604 school pupils aged 15–16. They found that 12.2% were ideators and 11.4% were enactors, with enactors differing significantly from ideators in terms of exposure to self-harm amongst family and friends, as well as impulsivity.

Online communities can significantly influence self-harm behaviours, both positively and negatively (House, 2020). These communities can provide support, understanding, and a sense of belonging for individuals struggling with self-harm, helping to reduce feelings of isolation. However, they can also normalise and even encourage self-harm through the sharing of graphic content and harmful advice. Research has shown that exposure to online content relating to self-harm can lead to an increase in self-harming behaviours, particularly among adolescents (Jenson et al., 2022; Marchant et al., 2017; Susi et al., 2023). To manage this risk, various strategies have been implemented, such as the introduction of psycho-educational prevention programmes in schools, stricter regulations for social media platforms, and the promotion of positive online behaviours. Major social media platforms like Tumblr, Pinterest, Instagram, and Facebook have responded to concerns by implementing policies that restrict or ban self-harm content and provide links to counselling and prevention resources (Samaritans, 2020). These measures aim to mitigate the negative impact of online communities while leveraging their potential for support and outreach.

Media guidelines for reporting self-harm and suicide are designed to minimise the risk of contagion and ensure responsible coverage. These guidelines emphasise the importance of avoiding sensationalism, providing accurate information, and including resources for those in need. For instance, the World Health Organization (WHO, 2025) advises against detailed descriptions of methods used in self-harm or suicide, as well as avoiding repetitive or prominent coverage of such incidents. The Samaritans' media guidelines recommend not disclosing the contents of suicide notes and avoiding the use of language that normalises or glamorises self-harm (Samaritans, ND).

Additionally, NICE highlights the need for multi-agency suicide prevention partnerships to encourage journalists and editors to follow best practices when reporting on suicide and self-harm (NICE, 2019). These measures aim to reduce the risk of imitation and provide support to vulnerable individuals.

Supporting People Immediately after Self-Harm

There is not one recommended model of care following incidents of self-harm (NICE, 2022a). If someone attends a healthcare setting and an assessment can be carried out, it is recommended that a mental health professional assesses and completes the care plan with the individual (NICE, 2022a). For example, in a general hospital, this may be someone from the mental health liaison team, or within a GP setting, it could be a specialist nurse. A person-centred psychosocial assessment with a care plan is often the most effective immediate intervention (NICE, 2022). This plan should be collaboratively created with the individual and include information about the frequency of aftercare, what this will look like, and its purpose, as well as who will be providing this care and support.

There are a number of reasons why patients may not receive a psychosocial assessment. These can include the patient feeling unable to ask or their refusing one due to previous negative experiences, or a patient may feel unable to remain in the emergency department due to feeling either psychologically or physically unsafe. People may not be offered an assessment or referred for one due to perceptions within the healthcare team that they attend regularly and that nothing has changed, or that a referral is not needed (Quinlivan et al., 2021).

Immediately following self-harm, research suggests people might feel guilty and ashamed when seeking help (Owens et al., 2018; O'Keeffe et al., 2021). Professionals may inadvertently increase these feelings while offering the care and treatment needed by making invalidating statements or suggesting that they do not want the individual to return following this episode. Validating and understanding someone's experience can lead to a much more positive outcome (O'Keeffe et al., 2021; Quinlivan et al., 2022). Similarly, O'Keeffe et al. (2021) found that spending time building rapport, listening to, and understanding the patient's needs, all help to improve their experiences and outcomes following self-harm, often leading to the person feeling safer. Understanding the functions of self-injurious actions, validating these, and then going on to create a supportive safety plan are all likely to lead to more positive outcomes for patients in the long term (O'Keeffe et al., 2021).

When planning treatment steps following an episode of self-harm, it's crucial to adopt a person-centred and strengths-focused approach (NICE, 2022). This may involve offering Cognitive Behavioural Therapy (CBT) for self-harm or other therapeutic interventions tailored to individual needs.

Challenges for the Person Seeking Help

One significant challenge faced by people who self-harm is the lack of continuity of care (NICE, 2022a) and the provision of limited services (O'Keeffe et al., 2021). Lack of follow-up support can increase the risk of repeated episodes of self-harm. Consequently, individuals often only receive support services when a crisis or self-harm incident has already occurred (O'Keeffe et al., 2021). Addressing these gaps in care and providing consistent, proactive support can help reduce the likelihood of recurring self-harming actions and improve overall outcomes.

With the above in mind, if someone is presenting to you following an episode of self-harm, then it is recommended to:

1. Provide appropriate physical health care and treatment for the injury.

2. If a mental health professional is available to complete a psychosocial assessment and care plan, then a referral (with the patient's knowledge and consent) can be made to them to request swift completion of this.

3. Care and safety plans should be created collaboratively with the person to support them to recognise their coping strategies and identify potential risks, alongside additional ways of accessing support.

4. When completing a risk assessment, risk should not be logged as low, medium, or high risk. Instead, a description should be provided of the risks (NICE, 2022). Similarly, NICE does not recommend the use of risk assessment tools.

5. Time spent understanding the reasons for and purpose behind the current self-harm can lead to more positive experiences for patients and service users. Similarly, positive experiences are more likely where understanding is demonstrated that the person may be feeling shame and guilt for attending hospital, and where care is taken to avoid inadvertently increasing these emotions, which could in turn increase the distress felt and potentially increase future risks.

6. Depending on your work environment, it is appropriate to remove items that could potentially be used to self-harm further (NICE, 2022). An example of this could be removing sharp objects from rooms if individuals are admitted to a hospital. Reducing access to the means can at times reduce the risk of repeated self-harm during admissions (NICE, 2022).

Tools for Now: Small Changes That Can Make a Big Difference

There are several ways in which you can support a patient or service user who is at risk of self-harming. These include a range of approaches to supporting the person to manage strong feelings and any urges to self-injure that are associated with these.

As a healthcare practitioner, you are likely to encounter individuals who report experiencing urges to self-harm. Sophie, in the case study, shares that she continues to struggle with strong urges to self-harm at times and feels unable to discuss these experiences openly. People may describe strong thoughts or desires to self-harm for a variety of reasons, whether they are currently self-harming, or have a history of self-harm. It is crucial to support and recognise the challenges involved in managing these urges.

One practice to help us understand what it feels like to manage urges is as follows:

- Set a timer for five minutes. During this time, sit completely still, with no fidgeting, no swallowing, no looking around.
- You can breathe and blink, but try to rest your eyes on one spot ahead of you and notice how it feels to resist all other movements until the timer sounds.

Many of us may not have had the experience of resisting urges, and it is important to recognise the challenge involved in asking someone to resist an urge or a compulsive behaviour. This short exercise can highlight how uncomfortable it can be to resist urges, even when we are feeling calm. Adding an element of distress would compound the challenge, yet we ask individuals experiencing urges to tolerate them for hours, sometimes days, before they are able to see a specialist practitioner.

Reflect on what you noticed while completing the urge resistance exercise above. Identify anything that helped you resist the urge to move, look around, or fidget. There may also have been things that made it harder to stay still. Take a moment to reflect on the huge challenge faced by patients and service users when they are expected to resist urges to self-harm in the context of overwhelmingly strong feelings that they long to reduce.

Supporting People to Manage Urges

One way to support individuals in managing their urges to self-harm is to help them safely dispose of items they might use for self-injury if they are having specific thoughts. For example, they may be willing to surrender additional medications or alcohol and to dispose of sharp objects. Doing this can help maintain their safety in the short term (NICE, 2022). It is essential to approach this process in a supportive and validating manner, rather than removing items without the person's consent or understanding. Conversations might include asking whether they are willing to dispose of these items and, if they agree, assisting them in planning and carrying out this process. If they are hesitant, looking for ways of understanding the reasons for this and identifying any barriers with them can be useful ways of providing further support (Ahmed et al., 2024).

Tolerating urges can be challenging, but Dialectical Behaviour Therapy (DBT) offers some specific skills that can be quickly taught and are simple to implement (Linehan, 2015).

TIP the Temperature

One such skill is TIP, also known as TIP the temperature (Linehan, 2015), which is related to the suite of TIPP skills identified in Chapter 2. TIP rapidly reduces emotional arousal and is particularly helpful for those feeling angry, anxious, struggling to sleep, or experiencing dissociation. It works by recreating the "dive reflex" to reduce heart rate.

To teach TIP, encourage individuals to run cold tap water into a sink or bowl. They should then bend over, hold their breath, and submerge their face (up to the temples) in the water for 30–60 seconds. Generally, the longer the immersion, the more effective this is, and they can take breaths and resubmerge as needed. Alternatively, they can use a bag filled with cold water and hold it to their cheeks if they prefer not to submerge their face. The process remains the same: bending over and holding their breath. Some people find that simply bending over, holding their breath, and splashing cold water on their face can be helpful, which may be more practical in public places.

There are precautions to consider with TIP. Due to the rapid slowing of the heart rate, individuals with heart problems, those on medications that reduce heart rate, or those with anorexia or bulimia nervosa should consult a medical professional to ensure it is safe for them. The effects of TIP are short-lived, so while it is helpful in the moment, intense emotions can resurface if the underlying problem is not addressed, or if other techniques are not also used. There is some evidence that cold-water therapy, such as cold showers, facial immersion, or cold-water swims, can also help reduce panic and depressive symptoms, though further research is needed (Carona and Marques, 2023).

Distraction

Distraction techniques, as highlighted by Linehan (2015), can be useful in managing urges and preventing immediate actions. Distraction is a strategy that many professionals have encouraged (Nawaz et al., 2021). However, incorrect teaching of these skills can potentially lead to increased frustration and disappointment for patients and service users.

It is important to remember that distraction will not solve patients' underlying problems. Therefore, it is essential to explain that distraction is a short-term measure that might provide a temporary break from the intensity of their experiences. Coaching is a vital strategy to adopt when encouraging people to use distraction, as it increases the likelihood that people will understand the purpose of and be willing to attempt using the tools. A common complaint in health services is that people are told to have a cup of tea, take a walk, or have a bath when they are in an acute emotional and mental health crisis. While these are examples of distraction, they are often presented as solutions to the problem of having an urge to self-harm, rather than as tools that can help to reduce emotional intensity, which in turn supports the patient in addressing the underlying issue.

Some effective distraction techniques to share for short-term relief include engaging in activities the person enjoys (such as listening to music, watching television, or interacting with a pet), helping others in ways that give them a sense of contribution, engaging in cognitive tasks (for example, counting games, crosswords, and puzzles), and using different sensations (for instance, a hot or cold shower, melting ice, and eating something spicy) (Linehan, 2015).

Self-Soothing

Self-soothing using sensory experiences can help reduce vulnerability to intense emotions and improve pain tolerance (Linehan, 2015). This technique focuses on being kind, comforting, and gentle towards oneself, a concept many patients find exceptionally challenging. Individuals can use the senses of sight, hearing, smell, taste, and touch to self-soothe. Examples include eating favourite foods, using a weighted blanket, watching clouds or stars, listening to soothing music or bird song, spending time at the beach or near water, and engaging in self-care routines such as applying skin cream or moisturiser. Self-soothing is unique to each person, and what each person finds soothing will vary. It is important to share ideas with patients while encouraging them to think about what they might personally find soothing. As with distraction, this is not intended to solve the underlying problem, but it does give the person a way of moving beyond that specific moment of intense and unbearable emotions.

Reducing and Managing Self-Harm: Understanding Specialist Interventions

A longer-term goal is to replace self-harm with more adaptive coping strategies. When asked, patients often express that they do not want to self-harm, but they can recognise the role self-harm plays in their lives (Woodley et al., 2021). As individuals learn and practice alternative approaches to coping, it is essential that they are supported consistently during each interaction with healthcare practitioners. Whether patients are receiving help from mental health professionals or independently learning new tools, we can assist them in integrating these strategies into their lives.

The NICE (2022) guidelines recommend treating co-existing conditions that may contribute to self-harming actions and urges. Alongside or following this treatment, it is advised to offer patients CBT-informed therapy, which could include CBT, DBT, problem-solving therapy, or other approaches. Westad et al. (2021) found that for individuals undergoing DBT, it took an average of 15.5 weeks for self-harming behaviours to cease. This underscores the importance of patience and long-term support, as therapy may take time to be effective while changes are being implemented.

In conjunction with structured therapy, safety planning and harm minimisation strategies are recommended to help keep individuals safe while they access these treatments. These combined efforts can provide a comprehensive approach to managing and reducing self-harm.

Summary of Learning Points

This chapter has explored the following theoretical and practical approaches to understanding non-suicidal self-harm:

- There are numerous reasons why someone may self-harm, and it is important that we work in ways that help us to understand these.
- Self-harm can increase if a person has close friends who also self-harm, or if people they know more generally do, as well as through social groups, or via social media, through which contagion can occur.
- Immediately following self-harm, a psychosocial care and safety plan is required, along with any physical treatment needed.
- There are several tools we can teach to patients who are likely to help them to manage their urges to self-harm in the short term.
- Specialist treatments are available for the longer term, including CBT and problem-solving approaches.

Questions for Reflection and Discussion

1. Although the functions of self-harm vary between and within individuals, what sorts of difficulties might it indicate are occurring, particularly around their underlying needs or emotional states?

2. How might harm minimisation approaches differ for various age groups or types of self-harm?

3. Identify ways in which the need to conduct a thorough risk assessment can be effectively balanced with the potential for causing distress or exacerbating stigma.

4. How can we ensure that our support is continuous and adaptive to the changing needs of individuals who self-harm?

5. In your role, how might you work in ways that complement the work of specialist practitioners to provide holistic care for individuals who self-harm?

Recommended Follow-up Reading

Hetrick, S.E., Subasinghe, A., Anglin, K., Hart, L., Morgan, A. and Robinson, J. (2020). Understanding the needs of young people who engage in self-harm: A qualitative investigation. *Frontiers in Psychology.* 10: 2916.

House, A. (2019). *Understanding and Responding to Self-Harm: The One Stop Guide: Practical Advice for Anybody Affected by Self-Harm.* London: Profile Books.

Linehan, M. (2015). *DBT Skills Training Manual.* (2nd ed). New York: Guilford Press.

Norman, H., Marzano, L., Oskis, A. and Coulson, M. (2022). "My heart and my brain is what's bleeding, these are just cuts." An interpretative phenomenological analysis of young women's experiences of self-harm. *Frontiers in Psychiatry.* 13, Article 914109: 1–7.

Denipitiya, T., Schlösser, A. and Bell, J. (2025). Mental health professionals' views on the influence of media on self-harm in young people: A critical discourse analysis. *Healthcare.* 13(14), 1640: 1–17.

References

Ahmed, N., Reynolds, L., Barlow, S., Mulligan, K., Drey, N. and Simpson, A. (2024). Barriers and enablers to shared decision-making in assessment and management of risk: A qualitative interview study with people using mental health services. *PLoS Mental Health.* 1(6): e0000157.

Bandura, A. (1977). *Social Learning Theory.* Englewood Cliffs: Prentice Hall.

Berger, E., Hasking, P. and Reupert, A. (2014). "We're working in the dark here": Education needs of teachers and school staff regarding student self-injury. *Journal of School Mental Health.* 6: 201–212.

Blasco-Frontecilla, H., Fernandez-Fernandez, R., Colino, L., Fajardo, L., Pergeguer-Barrio, R. and de Leon, J. (2016). The addictive model of self-harming (non-suicidal and suicidal) behaviour. *Frontiers in Psychiatry.* 7, Article 8:1–7.

Brown, M.Z., Comtois, K.A. and Linehan, M.M. (2002). Reasons for suicide attempts and nonsuicidal self-injury in women with borderline personality disorder. *Journal of Abnormal Psychology.* 111: 198–202.

Carona, C. and Marques, S. (2023). Beyond the cold baths: Contemporary applications of cold-water immersion in the treatment of clinical depression and anxiety. *BJPsych Advances.* 30(5): 271–273.

Chan, M.K.Y., Bhatti, H., Meader, N., Stockton, S., Evans, J., O'Connor, R.C., Kapur, N. and Kendall, T. (2018). Predicting suicide following self-harm: Systematic review of risk factors and risk scales. *The British Journal of Psychology.* 209(4): 277–283.

Christakis, N.A. and Fowler, J.H. (2013). Social contagion theory: Examining dynamic social networks and human behavior. *Statistics in Medicine.* 32(4): 556–577.

D'Agostino, A., Covanti, S., Rossi Monti, M. and Starcevic, V. (2017). Reconsidering emotion dysregulation. *Psychiatric Quarterly*. 88(4): 807–825.

Doyle, L., Sheridan, A. and Treacy, M.P. (2015). Self-harm in young people: Prevalence, associated factors, and help-seeking in school-going adolescents. *International Journal of Mental Health Nursing*. 24(6): 485–494.

Doyle, L., Sheridan, A. and Treacy, M.P. (2017). Motivations for adolescent self-harm and the implications for mental health nurses. *Journal of Psychiatric and Mental Health Nursing*. 24: 134–142.

Edwards, S.D. and Hewitt, J. (2011). Can supervising self-harm be part of ethical nursing practice? *Nursing Ethics*. 18(1): 79–87.

Hetrick, S.E., Subasinghe, A., Anglin, K., Hart, L., Morgan, A. and Robinson, J. (2020). Understanding the needs of young people who engage in self-harm: A qualitative investigation. *Frontiers in Psychology*. 10: 2916.

Himber, J. (1994). Blood rituals: Self-cutting in female psychiatric inpatients. *Psychotherapy*. 31: 620–631.

Himelein-Wachowiak, M., Giorgi, S., Kwarteng, A., Schriefer, D., Smitterberg, C., Yadeta, K., Bragard, E., Devoto, A., Ungar, L. and Curtis, B. (2022). Getting "clean" from nonsuicidal self-injury: Experiences of addition on the subreddit r/selfharm. *Journal of Behavioral Addictions*. 11(1): 128–139.

Hitchens, D., Boyda, D. and McFeeters, D. (2019). The role of Stressful Life Events and Emotion Regulation in Self-harm. *Conference: University of Wolverhampton Annual Research Conference*, Wolverhampton. Available online at: https://www.researchgate.net/publication/334654569_The_Role_of_Stressful_Life_Events_and_Emotion_Regulation_in_Self-Harm. [Accessed 2nd March 2025].

House, A. (2020). Social media, self-harm and suicide. *BJPsych Bulletin*. 44(4): 131–133.

Jenson, M.E., Vinberg, M., Andreasson, K., Klausen, J., Joergensen, K. and Nordentoft, M. (2022). Digital self-harm – social media and its impact on non-suicidal self-injury and suicidal behaviour. A longitudinal mixed method study. *European Psychiatry*. 65 (1): s341–s342.

Klonsky, E.D. (2007). The functions of deliberate self-injury: A review of the evidence. *Clinical Psychology Review*. 27(2): 226–239.

Linehan, M. (1993). *Cognitive-Behavioural Treatment for Borderline Personality Disorder*. New York: Guilford Press.

Linehan, M. (2015). *DBT Skills Training Manual*. (2nd ed). New York: Guilford Press.

Marchant, A., Hawton, K., Stewart, K., Montgomery, P., Singaravelu, V., Lloyd, K., Purdy, N., Daine, K. and John, A. (2017). A systematic review of the relationship between internet use, self-harm and suicidal behaviour in young people: The good, the bad and the unknown. *PLoS ONE*. 13(3): e0193937.

McManus, S., Bebbington, P., Jenkins, R. and Brugha, T. (eds.) (2016). Adult psychiatric morbidity survey: Survey of mental health and wellbeing, England (2014). Available online at: https://webarchive.nationalarchives.gov.uk/ukgwa/20180328140249/https://digital.nhs.uk/catalogue/PUB21748. [Accessed 2nd March 2025].

Nawaz, R.F., Reen, G., Bloodworth, N., Maughan, D. and Vincent, C. (2021). Interventions to reduce self-harm on in-patient wards: Systematic review. *BJPsych Open*. 7(3): e80, 1–9.

NICE (2019). Suicide prevention: Quality standard [QS189]. Quality statement 3: Media reporting. Available online at: https://www.nice.org.uk/guidance/qs189/chapter/Quality-statement-3-Media-reporting?form=MG0AV3&form=MG0AV3. [Accessed 2nd March 2025].

NICE (2022). Self-harm: Assessment, management and preventing recurrence. *NICE Guideline [NG225]*. Available online at: https://www.nice.org.uk/guidance/ng225%20accessed%2018th%20Jan%202025. [Accessed 2nd March 2025].

NICE (2022a). Self-harm: Assessment, management and preventing recurrence: Evidence reviews for models of care for people who have self-harmed. *NICE Guideline [NG225]*. Available online at: https://www.nice.org.uk/guidance/ng225/evidence/t-models-of-care-for-people-who-have-selfharmed-pdf-403069580857. [Accessed 2nd March 2025].

Nixon, M.K., Cloutier, P.F. and Aggarwal, S. (2002). Affect regulation and addictive aspects of repetitive self-injury in hospitalized adolescents. *Journal of the American Academy of Child and Adolescent Psychiatry*. 41: 1333–1341.

Nock, M.K. (2012). Future directions for the study of suicide and self-injury. *Journal of Clinical Child and Adolescent Psychology*. 41(2): 255–259.

O'Connor, R.C., Rasmussen, S. and Hawton, K. (2012). Distinguishing adolescents who think about self-harm from those who engage in self-harm. *British Journal of Psychiatry*. 200(4): 330–335.

O'Keeffe, S., Suzuki, M., Ryan, M., Hunter, J. and McCabe, R. (2021). Experiences of care for self-harm in the emergency department: Comparison of the perspectives of patients, carers and practitioners. *BJPsych Open*. 7: e175.

Owens, C., Hansford, L., Sharkey, S. and Ford, T. (2018). Needs and fears of young people presenting at accident and emergency and emergency department following an act of self-harm: Secondary analysis of qualitative data. *The British Journal of Psychiatry*. 208(3): 286–291.

Quinlivan, L.M., Gorman, L., Littlewood, D.L., Monaghan, E., Barlow, S.J., Campbell, S.M., Webb, R.T. and Kapur, N. (2021). 'Relieved to be seen'- patient and carer experiences of psychosocial assessment in the emergency department following self-harm: Qualitative analysis of 102 free-text survey responses. *BMJ Open*. 11: e044434.

Quinlivan, L.M., Gorman, L., Littlewood, D.L., Monaghan, E., Barlow, S.J., Campbell, S.M., Webb, R.T. and Kapur, N. (2022). 'Wasn't offered one, too poorly to ask for one'- reasons why some patients do not receive a psychosocial assessment following self-harm: Qualitative patient and carer survey. *Australian and New Zealand Journal of Psychiatry*. 56(4): 398–407.

Riggio, R.E., and Riggio, C.R. (2023). *Social contagion*. In S. Howard, H.S. Friedman and C.H. Markey (Eds.), *Encyclopaedia of Mental Health* (3rd ed). Oxford: Academic Press. V3-270–V3-273

Rogier, G., Petrocchi, C., D'aguanno, M. and Velotti, P. (2020). Self-harm and attachment in adolescents: What is the role of emotion dysregulation. *European Psychiatry*. 41(1): S222.

Sadath, A., Kavalidou, K., McMahon, E., Malone, K. and McLoughlin, A. (2024). Associations between humiliation, shame, self-harm and suicidality among adolescents and young adults: A systematic review. *PLoS ONE*. 19(2): 1–32.

Samaritans (2020). Managing self-harm and suicide content online: Guidelines for sites and platforms hosting user-generated content. Available online at: https://media.samaritans.org/documents/Online_Harms_guidelines_FINAL_1.pdf. 1–32. [Accessed 2nd March 2025].

Samaritans (ND). Samaritans' media guidelines. Available online at: https://www.samaritans.org/about-samaritans/media-guidelines/. [Accessed 2nd March 2025].

Susi, K., Glover-Ford, F., Stewart, A., Knowles Bevis, R. and Hawton, K. (2023). Research review: Viewing self-harm images on the internet and social media platforms: Systematic review of the impact and associated psychological mechanisms. *The Journal of Child Psychology and Psychiatry*. 64(8): 1115–1139.

Suyemoto, K.L. (1998). The functions of self-mutilation. *Clinical Psychology Reviews*. 18: 531–554.

Wang, L., Zou, H.O., Qu, Y.H., Hong, J.F. and Chen, J. (2025). The role of pain and blood simulation of nonsuicidal self-injury in emotion regulation among adolescents with depression based on the principle of harm reduction: An experimental study. *Behavior Therapy*. 56(3): 543–554.

Weinberg, A. and Klonsky, E.D. (2012). The effects of self-injury on acute negative arousal: A laboratory simulation. *Motivation and Emotion*. 36: 242–254.

Westad, Y.A.S., Hagen, K., Jonsbu, E. and Solem, S. (2021). Cessation of deliberate self-harm behaviour in patients with borderline personality traits treated with outpatient dialectical behaviour therapy. *Frontiers Psychology* 12: 578230.

Wester, K.L., Morris, C.W. and Williams, B. (2018). Nonsuicidal self-injury in the schools: A tiered prevention approach for reducing social contagion. *Professional School Counselling*. 21(1): 142–151.

WHO (2019). Self-harm and suicide. Available online at: https://www.who.int/teams/mental-health-and-substance-use/treatment-care/mental-health-gap-action-programme/evidence-centre/self-harm-and-suicide. [Accessed 2nd March 2025].

WHO (2025). Interact with media for responsible reporting of suicide. Available online at: https://www.who.int/initiatives/live-life-initiative-for-suicide-prevention/interact-with-media-for-responsible-reporting-of-suicide?form=MG0AV3&form=MG0AV3. [Accessed 2nd March 2025].

Wolff, J.C., Thompson, E., Thomas, S.A., Nesi, J., Bettis, A.H., Ransford, B., Scopelliti, K., Frazier, E.A. and Liu, R.T. (2019). Emotion dysregulation and non-suicidal self-injury: A systematic review and meta-analysis. *European Psychiatry*. 59: 25–36.

Wood, A. (2009). Self-harm in adolescents. *Advances in Psychiatric Treatment*. 15(6): 434–441.

Woodley, S., Hodge, S., Jones, K. and Holding, A. (2021). How individuals who self-harm manage their own risk - 'I cope because I self-harm, and I can cope with my self-harm'. *Psychological Reports*. 124(5): 1998–2017.

You, J., Lin, M.P., Fu, K. and Leung, F. (2013). The best friend and friendship group influence on adolescent nonsuicidal self-injury. *Journal of Abnormal Child Psychology*. 41: 993–1004.

5 Supporting People to Manage Suicidal Thoughts and Feelings

Hannah Bailey

Case Study

Jack's Story

I have struggled with depression throughout my life. Often, I would notice that I was getting more irritable and isolating myself from family and friends. Sometimes, I would have dark thoughts, but I always managed to push them aside. I can't recall if I mentioned these to my GP when I had my antidepressants reviewed.

During a low period, my wife told me she wasn't happy and wanted to separate. She asked me to move out in the next six weeks. We had been together for 30 years and I was utterly devastated. I had thoughts about ending my life and how I might go about this. I thought about how I might be able to make it look like an accident, so that it wouldn't upset the children so much.

I woke up exhausted every day. I hated asking my wife, but we agreed I would stay a little longer. I went to the GP, who referred me for therapy and reminded me it was normal to feel low during a relationship breakdown. I wasn't sure it was normal to have thoughts about suicide, but they didn't ask about them. I was too embarrassed to tell anyone about how I felt, and I was worried they would tell my work or lock me up in a hospital, so I didn't say anything. I was providing for my children and their needs, just focussing on them, as I couldn't do anything for my own future.

DOI: 10.4324/9781003635611-6

A restructure was announced at work. All I could think was that I had lost my family, my home, and now my job as well. Hearing this news, I decided that the time had come and that I was going to end my life. I couldn't face finding another job and I wasn't going to get my family into debt by taking money from them. They didn't need me as a financial burden too. I left work early and, on my way home, stopped at all shops I saw and bought as many tablets as I could, as well as some alcohol.

My wife found me in the bathroom, when she got home from work. I remember waking up in the hospital on a drip. When I was well enough, I was assessed by a nurse from the mental health liaison team. I told her I didn't want help and that I didn't want to talk about what was happening. I still wanted to end my life, though I had no intention of telling her. She was concerned about my unwillingness to talk to her, and I was admitted to hospital for assessment under Section 2 of The Mental Health Act.

On the ward, I remained low for quite some time. Medication helped, along with support from staff who took time to be with me. Very slowly, things began to improve, and after a few months of learning some tools and techniques to manage my mood and thoughts, I was discharged from the hospital.

I had support for quite a while from the Home Treatment Team and went on to receive treatment from the Community Mental Health Team. They helped me continue to learn ways of coping with stressful life events, to rebuild my life, and to find reasons to stay alive. They also helped me make sense of my separation and supported me to access employment and housing specialists. I really felt listened to. This made a big difference as I didn't have to bottle everything up inside myself. It felt as though I could work towards having some kind of future life.

Introduction

Approximately, one in five people will experience suicidal thoughts and feelings in their life and 1 in 15 people will attempt suicide (McManus et al., 2016; Iob et al., 2020; Samaritans, 2024). Following suicide attempts, only about 50% of people will seek help (McManus et al., 2016). Wherever we work in healthcare, we are likely to work with people who are experiencing suicidal thoughts as well as having opportunities to support people who have attempted suicide. Due to stigma, emotional ability, culture, shame, and embarrassment (Blanchard and Farber, 2018; Knapp, 2022), a large proportion of people who experience suicidal ideation do not seek help or support from health services (Hallford et al., 2023).

> ### Chapter Aims
>
> This chapter's focus is on suicidal ideation (thoughts) and feelings. It includes:
>
> - Developing an understanding of suicidal thoughts.
> - Understanding what can influence someone's risk of suicide.
> - How to assess suicidal risks and plan for safety.
> - Specialist interventions that may be available from mental health services.

Exploring Suicidal Thoughts

Of the people who have experienced suicidal thoughts, 50–60% of them have not shared these with anyone (Hallford et al., 2023), while a third of young people receiving therapy reported that they had not shared their suicidal thoughts with their therapist (McGillivray et al., 2022). However, when asked directly, only 21% of participants reported that they answered dishonestly or avoided the topic of suicidal thoughts and feelings (Blanchard and Farber, 2018). It is evident that while people may not feel able to volunteer this information, they are unlikely to hide it if asked, which highlights the importance of asking our patients and service users about the presence of any suicidal thoughts.

There are several reasons why patients may not feel comfortable disclosing suicidal ideation. This can include fear of punishment or adverse consequences (such as hospitalisation or the impact on their work), shame and stigma, or believing that no effective treatment exists, so nothing can be done to help them. In addition, the emotional pain caused by the disclosure itself can leave people feeling reluctant to discuss suicidal thoughts (Blanchard and Farber, 2018; Knapp, 2022; McGillivray et al., 2022). Knapp (2022) suggests several ways to support people to disclose suicidal thoughts and particularly highlights the importance of timing on the health practitioner's part. Waiting until a warm rapport has been established, and timing questions carefully are recommended ways of supporting disclosure, while a poorer therapeutic alliance is linked to non-disclosure (McGillivray et al., 2022).

The way we ask about suicidal thoughts can increase the likelihood of disclosure. For example, asking in an open way with a question such as "Are you having thoughts of suicide?" is more likely to support a patient to disclose than the more interrogative: "You aren't having any suicidal thoughts, are you?" which may come across as sounding accusational (McCabe et al., 2017; Knapp, 2022; Saini et al., 2024). From there, it is our task to gather additional information and details about these thoughts to support us in making safe and collaborative clinical decisions. When assessing and developing an understanding of suicidal thoughts and feelings, it is essential to ask for further details in the areas discussed in the following section on assessing suicidal thoughts. The information gathered will help guide the immediate next steps and subsequent safety planning.

Assessing Suicidal Thoughts

Active or Passive

Active thoughts are defined as thoughts of killing oneself, while passive thoughts involve having a desire for death. Both passive and active suicidal thoughts increase the risk of someone attempting suicide and can be present simultaneously (Wastler et al., 2022). These are illustrated in Table 5.1.

To help clarify whether thoughts are active or passive, we may ask questions such as: "Are your thoughts around wishing you could go to sleep and

Table 5.1 Examples of Active and Passive Suicidal Thoughts

Active	Passive
"I should kill myself". "I'm going to kill myself".	"I wish I hadn't been born". "I wish I could go to sleep and never wake up".

not wake up tomorrow, or more like planning to end your life in a particular way, or is it some of each?"

In our case study, Jack experiences occasional thoughts of suicide at first, though it is unclear whether these are active or passive. Although he does not explicitly state what kind of thoughts he is having, we can assume they have become active when he begins thinking about how he might end his life. This is something that would require further assessment and understanding.

Intent

Suicidal intent differs from suicidal ideation, and it is crucial to enquire about a person's intention to act on their thoughts (De Leo et al., 2021). This stage marks the beginning of forming plans and can lead to a suicide attempt, sometimes involving preparatory actions.

For example, people may share that they intend to buy medications to overdose with, or they may write a will, give away possessions, or engage in other preparatory acts. On the other hand, some people may state that they have active thoughts such as "I should take an overdose" but have no intention to buy or stockpile medications at that time.

When meeting people in healthcare environments, it is crucial to establish the intent behind episodes of self-harm. Suicidal intent at the point of self-harm is an indicator of future suicide risk (Harris et al., 2005). Even if the chosen method is unlikely to be fatal, or if the person independently sought support, in situations where the person believed their actions would lead to their death, we must treat what has taken place as seriously as if it had involved a method which would have been much more likely to be fatal (De Leo et al., 2021).

As an example, someone may believe that taking an additional Ibuprofen tablet will end their life and, after taking this overdose, will seek treatment from a hospital or GP. It is important to understand that this was a suicide attempt, which is just as serious as if they had taken an overdose involving multiple types and numbers of tablets.

Methods and Means

When developing an understanding of suicidal thoughts, it is important to ask about whether the individual you are speaking to has considered a method. Start the conversation with something like "If you were going to act on these thoughts, have you ever thought about what you would do?".

Often people may share one method, such as taking an overdose, but are likely to have thought about other ways, and so it is important to also ask about these (Marzano et al., 2021). Marzano et al. (2021) found that individuals often use a different method than the one they initially described. Therefore, asking about all the methods they have considered is crucial for assessing risks effectively.

In 2023, 58.8% of all deaths due to suicide were due to strangulation, hanging, and suffocation (Office for National Statistics, 2024). Understanding someone's thoughts is important to establish the level of immediate risk, as some methods are more dangerous, such as hanging or using a firearm (Cai et al., 2022).

We then need to ask if they have the means to act on the thoughts they have described. People may disclose plans to buy items on the way home, may share that they have what they need at home, or may say they have not yet taken any steps. This is where understanding other methods is important, as often, the choice of method is related to the accessibility of the means (Marzano et al., 2021).

For example, if someone states that they have thoughts of using a gun (method), we need to establish whether they have a gun at home (and therefore do have the means to harm themselves). We would also ask if they have thought of any other ways of carrying out their thoughts. If they state yes, and mention an overdose (method), we can then ask whether they have medications or other substances at home or plans to acquire them (the means). Depending on the responses, we would then make a clinical decision about the next best steps.

Removing access to both the methods and means of suicide is an effective way of preventing suicide (NICE, 2019; Royal College of Psychiatrists, 2020). Something for professionals to be aware of is, however, that changing someone's environment, for example, during an inpatient stay, may provide different or additional methods and means to act on suicidal ideation. With this in mind, it is important to consider the environment you work in and what actions and resources may be needed to support safety (NICE, 2019). This could be ensuring that there are no ligature points or making sure that sharps are always stored securely and kept out of the way.

Plans (Time)

Finally, we need to ask about specific plans and timeframes for acting. Plans include deciding how and when to act (De Leo et al., 2021). People may have a timeline and plan in place in their mind. For example, they may have thought of taking an overdose and plan on buying medications on the way home. However, that does not mean they will immediately take those tablets on their arrival home, as they may have other plans or steps to take prior to acting, such as waiting for a significant date, completing a will, or seeing friends. Understanding this timeline is essential for our clinical decision making.

Think about when Jack in our scenario developed a plan. He had spent time thinking about various methods, and yet the plan only firmly arose in his mind upon hearing about the potential loss of his job. It is quite likely that the plan to act on that day used a different method compared to what he had previously been considering.

In Cases of Uncertainty

If you have asked someone about suicidal thoughts and they have denied plans, thoughts, or intent, and yet you feel uncertain about their safety, there may be additional ways to support or encourage disclosure. Knapp (2022) found that asking twice in different ways can be helpful. For example, using a written questionnaire as well as an in-person interview can provide different responses and help communication become more open. There is further information about these types of written assessments later in this chapter, although they are secondary to clinical interviews.

As professionals, we need to remain calm, curious, and supportive (Knapp, 2022). People may not disclose their suicidal thoughts and intentions due to fear of judgement or punishment. Similarly, it may be helpful, to reduce someone's anxiety about disclosing, to highlight as part of the conversation that hospitalisation is only used as a last resort and that there are treatment options available at home (Blanchard and Faber, 2018; Knapp, 2022). To help reduce feelings of stigma, sharing how common suicidal thoughts can be may help reduce any shame associated with having them (Blanchard and Faber, 2018).

It is also quite likely that people with suicidal thoughts will be experiencing double stigma. Double stigma refers to experiencing stigma attached to both being mentally unwell and the stigma of suicide (Sheehan et al., 2017). This double stigma can reduce people's willingness to access care or to speak openly about what they are experiencing.

As part of establishing barriers to talking about suicidal thoughts, questions that can be asked are: "If you were experiencing suicidal thoughts, would you feel able to tell me?" or "Do you have any worries about sharing your symptoms with me?". If someone responds in a way that signals that there are barriers, this provides an opportunity to work on reducing these.

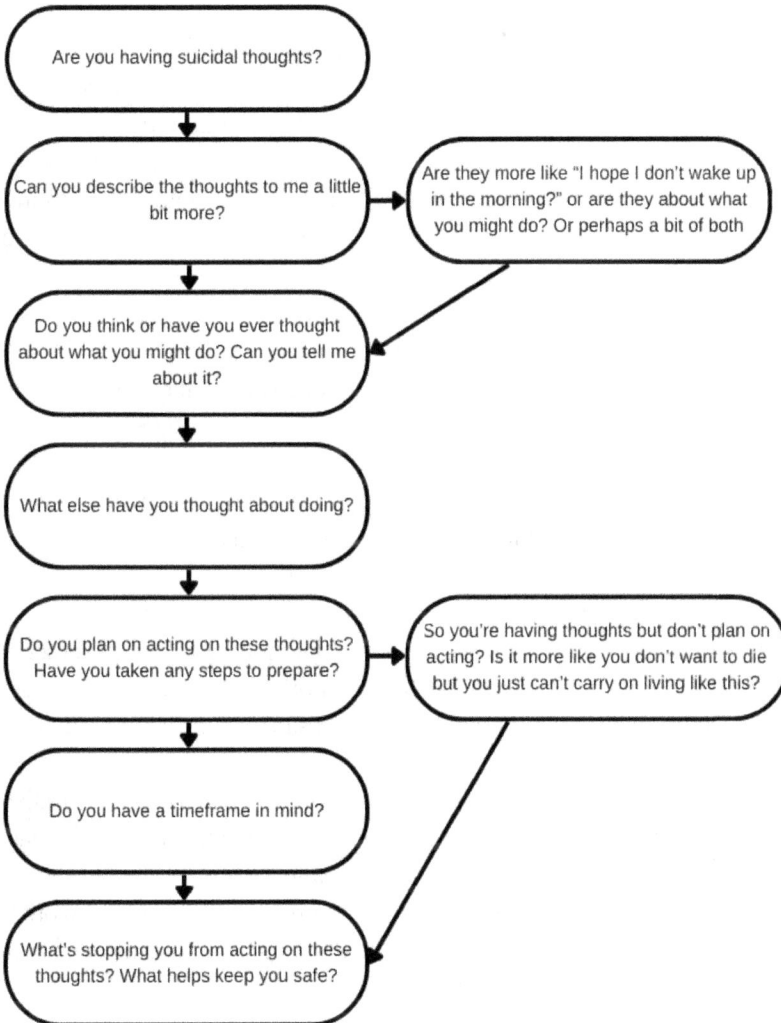

Are you having suicidal thoughts?

Can you describe the thoughts to me a little bit more?

Are they more like "I hope I don't wake up in the morning?" or are they about what you might do? Or perhaps a bit of both

Do you think or have you ever thought about what you might do? Can you tell me about it?

What else have you thought about doing?

Do you plan on acting on these thoughts? Have you taken any steps to prepare?

So you're having thoughts but don't plan on acting? Is it more like you don't want to die but you just can't carry on living like this?

Do you have a timeframe in mind?

What's stopping you from acting on these thoughts? What helps keep you safe?

Figure 5.1 The Process of Assessing Suicidal Thoughts here.

It is important to remember that even if people deny suicidal thoughts, they may still be at risk of dying by suicide (Royal College of Psychiatrists, 2020). Therefore, identifying risk factors can help us understand more and support us in seeking appropriate further help (Figure 5.1).

Risk Assessments and Planning for Safety

Identifying Risk Factors

To be clear, if it hasn't been clear elsewhere, it is essential that we ask about thoughts of suicide. Asking someone about suicide does not increase the risk of them acting upon their thoughts and can actually be a protective factor that reduces the risk of acting on those thoughts (Dazzi et al., 2014).

A range of risk factors exist, which may increase the potential of an individual acting on their suicidal thoughts. Some that stand out are outlined below:

- Living alone (McManus et al., 2016). It is important to ask our patients whether they are living alone if we are unaware of their current living situation.
- Being out of work (McManus et al., 2016).
- Being from a minority background (Royal College of Psychiatrists, 2020).
- Men, particularly middle-aged men, are more likely to die by suicide than women (Office for National Statistics, 2023).
- Being divorced or single (Office for National Statistics, 2023).
- A history of self-harm or mental health conditions (Favril et al., 2022).
- Chronic pain and long-term health conditions, alongside the person seeing themselves as a burden due to these disabilities (Cheatle, 2024).

Many of these risk factors are static, or stable, factors. Static factors are fixed and will not change, such as if someone has experienced abuse or has a history of suicide attempts. By contrast, stable factors are long-term and enduring but are not fixed, such as where a person has been out of work for a long time or has a long-term mental health diagnosis such as personality disorder (Bouch and Marshall, 2005).

Bouch and Marshall (2005) highlight that static and stable risks may provide an insight into understanding an individual's baseline risk of suicide, but they cannot capture the fluctuating circumstances and changes in risk associated with dynamic and future risks.

Dynamic risk factors fluctuate in duration and intensity and could include feelings of hopelessness or substance use, while future factors include aspects such as acquiring access to potential methods (Bouch and Marshall, 2005). Dynamic and future risk factors are likely to have been a precipitating factor leading to any current crisis.

Discussion about a person's current active or passive thoughts, plans, means, methods, and intent will support us to formulate our risk assessment with the outcomes of these questions guiding our decision making and care planning with the individual. Holding static, stable, dynamic, and future risk factors in our mind can also support us with decision making (Bouch and Marshall, 2005).

Risk Assessment Tools – Something to Be Aware Of

When discussing risk assessment in this section, we are referring to risk assessment tools, questionnaires, and paperwork that use an actuarial approach to assessing risk (Bouch and Marshall, 2005). Often, these risk tools will lead practitioners to describe someone as being at no, low, medium, or high risk. NICE (2022) state that this should not be used as a measure or way of describing someone's risk, and instead, we should describe the precise risks posed.

More structured and formalised risk assessments may help professionals in high stress situations feel more confident. However, NICE discourages their use as they do not align with best practice. Unfortunately, they continue to be used in some areas of practice, despite contradicting guidance (NICE, 2022; Fedorowicz et al., 2023).

As outlined at the start of this chapter, open questions are more likely to lead to honest and detailed responses (McCabe et al., 2017; Knapp, 2022; Saini et al., 2024). When using assessment tools, there is a chance that specific human factors leading to suicidal ideation are missed, which can prevent patients from expressing their unique experiences and may increase the risk of them feeling invalidated (Pompili, 2024).

Appropriate documentation needs to be completed to outline the clinical assessment, and a risk formulation must be completed by the clinician who met with the patient (NICE, 2022). This should be collaborative and outline the patient's current difficulties to support and create an appropriate care and treatment plan. This formulation will include historical factors (such as previous suicide attempts), recent problems, current strengths, and protective factors. Something to consider and acknowledge is that often a barrier to thorough and detailed risk assessments and formulations can be our working environments (Saini et al., 2024). This may include time constraints, the physical environment, or limited opportunities to build rapport with patients and service users.

Protective Factors

It is equally important to ask patients about their protective factors, which are defined as factors that reduce the likelihood of someone engaging in suicidal behaviour (McLean et al., 2008). These will be unique to individuals, and it is important not to make assumptions about protective factors. When asking about protective factors questions such as "What is stopping you from acting on the suicidal thoughts we spoke about earlier?" can be useful.

Some general protective factors suggested by research are outlined briefly below. There is limited research into protective factors, and so, it is essential we discuss what helps keep our individual patients safe when meeting with them and when completing assessments and safety plans:

- Positive self-perceptions (Bakken et al., 2024, 2025).
- Purpose in life (Ki et al., 2024).
- Coping strategies that are not based on emotion (Bakken et al., 2024).
- Being able to identify resources and strategies for resilience (Ki et al., 2024).
- Social connections and support (Ki et al., 2024).
- Hopefulness and feeling that there are reasons for living (McLean et al., 2008).

A key aspect to consider about protective factors when thinking about any risk is that they may not always be available, present, or consistent. For example, if someone describes their child as being a protective factor, we need to think about what happens when their child moves out, is away for the weekend, or the relationship is damaged or disrupted in some way. Similarly, if a partner is a protective factor, considering the effects of an argument can be key to understanding the inconsistent nature of some protective factors.

The risk and protective factors for Jack varied throughout his life and highlight how protective factors can quickly change. These are shown in Table 5.2.

Table 5.2 Jack's Risk and Protective Factors

Jack's risk factors	Jack's protective factors
• Male • Recent ending of a relationship • Uncertainty about work • Isolated from family and friends • History of depression • Experiencing suicidal ideation • Middle-aged	• Historically, providing for his family may have been included as a protective factor, but it is unlikely Jack would describe this now. • Historically, Jack may have described his relationship as a protective factor.

Tools for Now: Small Changes That Can Make a Big Difference

Safety Planning

Safety plans are co-produced with patients and require a warm, nonjudgemental, therapeutic relationship and compassionate approach (Royal College of Psychiatrists, 2020). Such plans include details of activities, coping strategies, and who to contact if the thoughts become worse or in situations where the person feels unable to maintain their safety (Royal College of Psychiatrists, 2020; NICE, 2022). These plans need to be individualised to the person we are working with and may include some basic steps for solving the problems the individual faces. Often people experiencing suicidal thoughts may not want to die but are unable to continue living with the extent of mental pain and emotional distress they are experiencing, and so suicide is perceived as providing a solution to this (Pompili, 2024).

Safety planning is an intervention that needs to be completed with anyone experiencing suicidal thoughts. The Royal College of Psychiatrists (2020) recommend that the following areas are considered in safety plans:

- Reasons for living and ideas for getting through difficult times. If you have completed pros and cons with someone, these may help guide this area of safety planning. If not, then it is worth discussing with someone what reasons they might have to live. These may include pets, friends and family, things that people enjoy doing, and plans that they may have previously mentioned looking forward to.
- Making the current situation safer. These are steps that the person can take to increase their own safety. It could include disposing of methods,

seeking support from helpful friends and family, or other steps that help someone increase their safety.

- Things to lift their mood. This is anything that might improve someone's mood. Support people to be as specific as possible; so, for example, rather than saying "watch television", be specific about exactly which programmes they might enjoy watching. It is important to explain that this, and the following areas of the plan, will help alleviate some of the pain in the short term. However, it should also be acknowledged that we understand these approaches will not solve the problems in the long term and that we therefore want to support them to gain the support to do that as well (Linehan, 2015).
- Things to calm their mood (anything relaxing). Like lifting their mood, this is thinking about what might help someone relax when their feelings are too much to manage. There may be some overlap of these two areas in terms of the strategies used.
- Distractions that can be used. Using distraction can be helpful to manage short-term crisis situations. It is important to remember that distraction does not solve the problems people are seeking help with (Linehan, 2015), but it can be helpful to manage the immediate urges that people may be experiencing.
- Additional sources of support. These can include professional sources of support, including emergency services and telephone numbers, as well as any informal supporters the person has.

Taking Time to Understand

Given the importance of establishing rapport and gathering details about people's thoughts, taking our time is essential in supporting this process. When people feel they have no other options available to them, suicide can offer a potential solution to the problems they are facing and can look like a way of escaping from and ending, intolerable circumstances, and suffering (Pompili, 2024). There is evidence that people who experience intense suicidal ideation or who act on suicidal thoughts have poorer problem-solving skills (Darvishi et al., 2023; Heapy et al., 2024). Suicide may seem to provide a solution for mental and physical health problems, financial worries, relationship difficulties, housing challenges, or any combination and number of situations, where more wide-ranging solutions cannot be envisioned.

Understanding the problems faced by our patients is a first step toward planning for safety in the long term.

Inviting people to talk about suicidal thoughts shows a willingness to begin to understand, as well as being essential for making an assessment and responding to the problems a person is facing. Talking is a starting point, which can bring about longer-term changes. The goal is to work with each person to change the reasons behind wanting to die and to address the factors causing life to feel unbearable. This is likely to involve bringing in additional support services.

As practitioners, we can work on several aspects to help us, and our patients and service users, to understand what may be contributing to suicidal thoughts and feelings and begin to support a more constructive approach to problem-solving.

Taking our time to explore the pros and cons (Linehan, 2015) of either acting on, or resisting acting on, suicidal thoughts may provide additional information about the person's situation. To complete a pros and cons chart with someone requires a trusting and therapeutic relationship, as it asks them to consider potentially painful reasons why they may or may not act on their thoughts.

An example of a pros and cons chart is provided in Table 5.3 with reference to Jack's situation.

Table 5.3 Example Pros and Cons of Acting on Suicidal Thoughts

	Pros	Cons
Acting on suicidal urges	No more worries about work or relationships. I won't have to find somewhere else to live. I won't be in pain anymore. I won't be a financial burden to my family.	If it doesn't work, I may be left in a worse state. If it doesn't work, my wife may stay because she feels guilty. If it works, my children will be impacted.
Resisting suicidal urges	I'll get to see my children grow up, maybe meet my grandchildren. I have things I would like to achieve still in life. My children won't be upset or hurt, suicide won't impact them and their lives. My wife won't be upset.	I will have to tolerate feeling terrible right now. I will have to find a new home and possibly a new job.

As you can see from Table 5.3, there are several pros and cons for Jack both if he acts and if he resists his urges. This helps to highlight some of the problems that suicide may solve for him, such as not having to find alternative employment and relieving his current emotional pain. Our task would be to support him to solve these problems in alternative ways. This is likely to require working with external agencies to support with housing, employment, and financial advice, alongside treatment for his ongoing depressive symptoms. It is likely that the required ongoing support will, in part, be offered by specialist services.

Suicidal Thoughts: Referral to Specialist Services

Referral criteria will differ from location to location around the UK, and different teams and services may be available in each area. However, if you are concerned for someone's welfare and they are experiencing suicidal thoughts, an onward referral is likely to be appropriate for longer-term support in managing these.

In a crisis, a referral to a Crisis Resolution and Home Treatment Team may be suitable as an alternative to hospital admission or for a more urgent mental health assessment to then support care planning. If someone has already acted on their thoughts and is seeking treatment, it is recommended that a referral is made for a psychosocial assessment by a mental health professional (NICE, 2022).

If someone is experiencing suicidal thoughts and feelings but does not have a plan, method, or intent in mind, then an onward referral to a Community Mental Health Team may be another option. This may be a slower referral, but it is likely to lead to a longer period of stabilisation and treatment rather than a brief period of intervention.

The decision around which team to refer to will be based on understanding the level of distress and whether this is currently increasing, alongside whether suicidal intent is increasing, and your own levels of concern (NICE, 2022).

Summary of Learning Points

This chapter has explored the following aspects of suicidal thoughts:

- Health practitioners have a duty to understand and assess suicidal thoughts.

- A thorough assessment can help with planning next steps in an individual's treatment plan.
- Understanding the reasons why someone may be experiencing suicidal thoughts can support healthcare practitioners to involve other agencies to support problem-solving.
- Safety planning is recommended for all those who are experiencing suicidal ideation.
- Onward referral to secondary mental health services can support follow-up.

Questions for Reflection and Discussion

1. Are you one of the 45% of people (Samaritans, 2024) who feel uncomfortable having a conversation about suicide? If so, what steps can you take to support you to have these difficult conversations in your practice?

2. At what points in Jack's story could the outcome have been different? Where could health professionals have intervened earlier and what warning signs were present?

3. If Jack had sought support earlier, what could that support have looked like?

4. Have you ever described someone as being at "no/low/medium/high risk" of suicide in documentation or to colleagues? How could you better describe the details about people's experiences and risks in the future?

5. Identify the difficulties and challenges associated with making a risk assessment in your setting. How could some of these challenges be overcome?

Recommended Follow-up Reading

4 Mental Health Ltd. (2025). Staying safe from suicidal thoughts. Available online at: https://stayingsafe.net/. [Accessed 21st August 2025].

Bouch, J. and Marshall, J.J. (2005). Suicide risk: Structured professional judgement. *Advances in Psychiatric Treatment*. 11(2): 84–91.

Kalashnikova, O., Leontiev, D., Rasskazova, E. and Taranenko, O. (2022). Meaning of life as a resource for coping with psychological crisis: Comparisons of suicidal and non-suicidal patients. *Frontiers in Psychology.* 13. 957782: 1–15.

Pompili, M. (2024). On mental pain and suicide risk in modern psychiatry. *Annals of General Psychiatry.* 23(1): 1–13.

Zheng, B., Zhu, N., Yu, M., Guan, Y., Zheng, Z., Deng, Y. and Jiang, Y. (2025). Single question for screening suicide risk in patients with cancer in nursing routine work: A retrospective cross-sectional study. *Journal of Advanced Nursing (John Wiley & Sons, Inc.).* 81(8): 4627–4643.

References

Bakken, V., Lydersen, S., Skokauskas, N., Sund, A.M. and Kaasbøll, J. (2024). Protective factors for suicidal ideation: A prospective study from adolescence to adulthood. *European Child & Adolescent Psychiatry.* 33: 3079–3089.

Bakken, V., Lydersen, S., Skokauskas, N., Sund, A.M. and Kaasbøll, J. (2025). Protective factors for suicidal ideation and suicide attempts in adolescence: A longitudinal population-based cohort study examining sex differences. *BMC Psychiatry.* 25: 106.

Blanchard, M. and Farber, B.A. (2018). "It is never okay to talk about suicide": Patients' reasons for concealing suicidal ideation in psychotherapy. *Psychotherapy Research.* 30(1): 124–136.

Bouch, J. and Marshall, J.J. (2005). Suicide risk: Structured professional judgement. *Advances in Psychiatric Treatment.* 11(2): 84–91.

Cai, Z., Junus, A., Chang, Q. and Yip, P.S.F. (2022). The lethality of suicide methods: A systematic review and meta-analysis. *Journal of Affective Disorders.* 300: 121–129.

Cheatle, M.D. (2024). Pain, substance use disorder and suicide: On the edge. *Current Addiction Reports.* 11: 809–817.

Darvishi, N., Farhadi, M., Azmi-Naei, B. and Poorolajal, J. (2023). The role of problem-solving skills in the prevention of suicidal behaviours: A systematic review and meta-analysis. *PLoS ONE.* 18(10): e0293620.

Dazzi, T., Gribble, R., Wessely, S. and Fear, N.T. (2014). Does asking about suicide and related behaviours induce suicidal ideation? What is the evidence? *Psychological Medicine.* 44(16): 3361–3363.

De Leo, D., Goodfellow, B., Silverman, M., Berman, A., Mann, J., Arensman, E., Hawton, K., Phillips, M.R., Vijayakumar, L., Andriessen, K., Chavez-Hernandez, A-M., Heisel, M. and Kolves, K. (2021). International study of definitions of English-language terms for suicidal behaviours: A survey exploring preferred terminology. *BMJ Open.* 11(2): e043409.

Favril, L., Yu, R., Uyar, A., Sharpe, M. and Fazel, S. (2022). Risk factors for suicide in adults: Systematic review and meta-analysis of psychological autopsy studies. *Evidence Based Mental Health.* 25: 148–155.

Fedorowicz, S., Dempsey, E.C., Ellis, N.J., Mulvey, O. and Gidlow, C.J. (2023). Quantitative content analysis of freedom of information requests examining the extent and variations of tools and training for conducting suicide risk assessments in NHS Trusts across England. *BMJ Open*. 26(13): e072004.

Hallford, D.J., Rusanov, D., Winestone, B., Kaplan, R., Fuller-Tyszkiewicz, M. and Melvin, G. (2023). Disclosure of suicidal ideation and behaviours: A systematic review and meta-analysis or prevalence. *Clinic Psychology Review*. 101: 102272.

Harris, L., Hawton, K. and Zahl, D. (2005). Value of measuring suicidal intent in the assessment of people attending hospital following self-poisoning or self-injury. *The British Journal of Psychiatry*. 186: 60–66.

Heapy, C., Haddock, G. and Pratt, D. (2024). The relationship between social problem-solving and suicidal ideation and behaviour in adults: A systematic review and meta-analysis. *Clinical Psychology: Science and Practice*. 31(4): 419–432.

Iob, E., Steptoe, A. and Fancourt, D. (2020). Abuse, self-harm and suicidal ideation in the UK during the CPVOD-19 pandemic. *The British Journal of Psychiatry*. 217: 543–546.

Ki, M., Lapierre, S., Gim, B., Hwang, M., Kang, M., Dargis, L., Jung, M., Koh, E.J. and Mishara, B. (2024). A systematic review of psychosocial protective factors against suicide and suicidality among older adults. *International Psychogeriatrics*. 36(5): 346–370.

Knapp, S. (2022). Six strategies to help reluctant patients to disclose their suicidal thoughts. *Practice Innovations*. 7(4): 293–302.

Linehan, M.M. (2015). *DBT Skills Training Manual*. (2nd ed). New York: The Guildford Press.

Marzano, L., Katsampa, D., Mackenzi, JM., Kruger, I., El-Gharbawi, N., Ffolkes-St-Helene, D., Mohiddin, H. and Fields, D. (2021). Patterns and motivations for method choices in suicidal thoughts and behaviour: Qualitative content analysis of a large online survey. *BJPsych Open*. 7: e60, 1–6.

McCabe, R., Sterno, I., Priebe, S. Barnes, R. and Byng, R. (2017). How do healthcare professionals interview patients to assess suicide risk? *BMC Psychiatry*. 17: 122.

McGillivray, L., Rheinberger, D., Wang, J., Burnett, A. and Torok, M. (2022). Non-disclosing youth: A cross sectional study to understand why young people do not disclose suicidal thoughts to their mental health professional. *BMC Psychiatry*. 22(1): 1–11.

McLean, J., Maxwell, M., Platt, S., Harris, F. and Jepson, R. (2008). Risk and protective factors for suicide and suicide behaviour: A literature review. *Scottish Government Social Research; Scottish Government*, Edinburgh. Available online at: https://dspace.stir.ac.uk/bitstream/1893/2206/1/Suicide%20review1.pdf. [Accessed 21st August 2025].

McManus, S., Bebbington, P., Jenkins, R. and Brugha, T. (eds.) (2016). Adult psychiatric morbidity survey: Survey of mental health and wellbeing, England 2014. Available online at: https://webarchive.nationalarchives.gov.uk/ukgwa/20180328140249/https://digital.nhs.uk/catalogue/PUB21748. [Accessed 5th January 2025].

NICE (2019). Suicide prevention. NICE quality standard QS189. Available online at: https://www.nice.org.uk/guidance/qs189/resources/suicide-prevention-pdf-7554 5729771461. [Accessed 28th February 2025].

NICE (2022). Self-harm: Assessment, management and preventing recurrence. *NICE Guideline NG225*. Available online at: https://www.nice.org.uk/guidance/ng225. [Accessed 28th February 2025].

Office for National Statistics (2023). Sociodemographic inequalities in suicides in England and Wales: 2011 to 2021. Available online at: https://www.ons.gov.uk/ peoplepopulationandcommunity/healthandsocialcare/healthinequalities/ bulletins/sociodemographicinequalitiesinsuicidesinenglandandwales/2011 to2021. [Accessed 28th February 2025].

Office for National Statistics (2024) Published 29th August 2024. Available onlineat:https://www.ons.gov.uk/peoplepopulationandcommunity/birthsdeathsand marriages/deaths/bulletins/suicidesintheunitedkingdom/2023#:~:text=There%20 were%206%2C069%20suicides%20registered,highest%20rate%20seen%20 since%201999. [Accessed 28th February 2025].

Pompili, M. (2024). On mental pain and suicide risk in modern psychiatry. *Annals of General Psychiatry*. 23(1): 1–13.

Royal College of Psychiatrists (2020). Self-harm and suicide in adults: Final report of the patient safety group. Available online at: https://www.rcpsych.ac.uk/docs/ default-source/improving-care/better-mh-policy/college-reports/college-report-cr229-self-harm-and-suicide.pdf?sfvrsn=b6fdf395_10. [Accessed 28th February 2025].

Saini, P., Hunt, A., Blaney, P. and Murray, A. (2024). Recognising and responding to suicide-risk factors in primary care: A scoping review. *Journal of Prevention*. 45: 727–750.

Samaritans (2024). Suicidal thoughts more common than many realise as new Samaritans survey reveals public attitudes to 'taboo' subject. Available online at: https://www.samaritans.org/news/suicidal-thoughts-more-common-than-many-realise-new-samaritans-survey-reveals/. [Accessed 15th August 2025].

Sheehan, L.L., Corrigan, P.W. and Al-Khouja, M.A. (2017). Stakeholder perspectives on the stigma of suicide attempt survivors. *Crisis: The Journal of Crisis Intervention and Suicide Prevention*. 38(2): 73–81.

Wastler, H.M., Khazem, L.R., Ammendola, E., Baker, J.C., Bauder, C.R., Tabares, J., Bryan, A.O., Szeto, E. and Bryan, C.J. (2022). An empirical investigation of the distinction between passive and active ideation: Understanding the latent structure of suicidal thought content. *Suicide and Life-Threatening Behavior*. 53: 219–226.

Reasons to Go On

6

Helping People Find Hope in a Crisis

Hannah Bailey and
Louise Cherrill

Case Study

Ella's Story

I don't remember the first time I had suicidal thoughts. I first went to get help from the GP as a teenager. My Mum took me because she was worried that I was falling into a bad crowd, taking drugs, and self-harming by cutting myself when I felt angry or sad. I found that cutting helped take those suicidal feelings away.

I kept doing what I thought I was meant to, having relationships, going to university, but it didn't solve the problems I was having and, if anything, created more. I struggled with my studies, and I went off sick. I just couldn't imagine finding a long-term job or a partner because my emotions were getting more intense.

I dropped out of university, my only real joy for a long time was my pet cat and when she died, life became even harder. I decided that I couldn't carry on living like this. It was just one grey day after another. I took an overdose and was admitted to the emergency department at the local hospital. I had panicked and called an ambulance after taking the tablets.

While I was in the hospital, I spoke to the Mental Health Liaison Team. The nurse there took time to listen to me and she said that she could understand why I had done what I had done, that it was me trying to solve a problem. She took time to listen and tried to help me think about what needed to happen next to help keep me safe. She offered to refer me on to the Community Mental Health Team (CMHT) for help.

DOI: 10.4324/9781003635611-7

> *We spoke about how it might take some time, but that life could be different if I was willing to be supported to find other ways of solving problems. I was informed the CMHT could help with problems I was facing emotionally and support me to access help from other services specialising in education, benefits, and employment.*
>
> *After a while, I started a therapy called Dialectical Behavioural Therapy (DBT). I was sceptical about it but also knew something had to change because life couldn't continue as it was. The therapists I worked with helped me understand what was important to me, something I'd never really been able to work out. They taught me how to build my life up around these things. With hindsight now, I can see I didn't actually want to die. At the time, my life was unbearable, chaotic, and full of suffering because I didn't know how to get what I needed and wanted from it. The team helped me learn how to manage my emotions so that they didn't keep getting in the way of the things that I would really like to do.*
>
> *It has been a few years since I finished my treatment and I now run my own dog walking business, something I'd never thought about doing before. I enjoy being out, seeing all the dogs, and feel proud that my clients trust me with caring for their pets.*

Introduction

Suicide, the act of intentionally causing one's own death or making attempts to do this, was considered a crime before the 1960s and was dealt with by the police (Millard, 2015). It is now recognised as a mental health emergency and is managed by healthcare professionals. Despite this change, the language used to describe suicide is still caught up in the historical legal framework. For example, within the phrase "commit suicide", the word *commit* refers semantically to an act that is illegal or immoral (Oxford University Press, 2024).

It is challenging to provide accurate suicide statistics for several reasons. These statistics are refreshed yearly or quarterly depending on the publisher, and because of the delay caused by analysis and publication, they are always slightly out of date. Sources where you can access this information (in its most up to date form) include the Healthcare Quality Improvement Partnership (2025), the Office for National Statistics (2024), and the Office for Health Improvement and Disparities (2025).

There has been some variation in the rates of suicide over the years, although these rates were stable at 10.7 per 100k deaths in 2021–2022, increasing to 11.4 per 100k in 2023, which is the highest rate since 1999 (Office for National Statistics, 2024). However, other elements of the data remain stable, including suspected suicides being higher in males (14.4 per 100k) than females (5 per 100k), the most at risk being those aged 45–64 (13.3 per 100k), and hanging, suffocation, or strangulation being the most common methods (55.2%) (Office for Health Improvement and Disparities, 2025).

Feeling suicidal, that is, having thoughts about not wanting to be alive anymore, is often the manifestation of someone attempting to solve a temporary problem with a permanent solution. These problems might include life events and difficult feelings or be symptomatic of mental illness. Seeking help for these feelings is inhibited by not feeling worthy of support, not knowing where to ask for it, and being fearful of an unhelpful response following disclosure (Barnett et al., 2024).

Working with suicidal people and managing deaths from completed suicides can be challenging. The internal and external investigatory process can suggest that perhaps prevention efforts (or the healthcare staff involved) have failed, which is not the case following deaths from other causes in healthcare. This can lead to risk-avoidant practice and a blame culture (Gibbons, 2024). Health practitioners rely on quantifying risk based on a series of factors (discussed in Chapter 5), and assurances from the patient that they will follow a self-rescue safety plan should they no longer be able to keep themselves or others safe. Hawton et al. (2022) provide a detailed discussion of why this method of risk assessment is not therapeutic and explore some alternatives that may be better.

Chapter Aims

This chapter will cover the following areas of theory and contemporary practice in relation to supporting people who are in mental health crisis:

- An introduction to the law and the legal complexities arising when working with suicidal individuals.
- An exploration of potential professional anxieties and how to manage these.

- Tools that can be used to help inspire hope for the future for patients and service users, including how having an understanding of personal values and goal setting can support a treatment plan.
- A brief overview of the emergency mental health care available.

Understanding the Law

There are several legal duties for us to understand in relation to suicide and caring for people who are experiencing suicidal ideation. This includes people who have plans or intent, or have acted upon suicidal thoughts and intent.

The Mental Health Act (MHA) (1983, as amended by the Mental Health Act 2007) can be used to detain someone who has a mental disorder in a hospital for a period of assessment or treatment, if it is in the interests of their own safety or the safety of others. This can occur following a MHA assessment in line with the Mental Health Act 1983 (as amended): Code of Practice (Department of Health, 2015), usually completed by an Approved Mental Health Professional and two Registered Medical Practitioners, who decide if the parameters for legal detention under the Act have been met.

A fundamental component of the provision of care as a health care professional is the need for informed consent. The Mental Capacity Act (MCA) (Department of Health, 2005) is clear that it must be assumed that people have the capacity to make decisions, including the right to make unwise decisions. This includes decisions about the care and treatment that we offer as healthcare professionals. If we have a reason to doubt the capacity (such as an impairment or disturbance in functioning to the mind or brain), then it is our task to determine the capacity by assessing the person's ability to understand, weigh up, and retain information about a decision and to then communicate their decision (Department of Health, 2005). Healthcare practitioners must take all reasonable measures to help the person to complete the steps for the assessment of capacity, such as using communication aids. It is important to remember that capacity is time- and decision-specific. Decision-specific refers to the idea that someone may have the capacity to choose the colour of the t-shirt they wish to wear or what they wish to eat for breakfast, but not where they would like to live (for example, at home versus in a supported living accommodation). Time-specific refers to the idea that the person may regain the capacity (such as in the case of lacking the capacity due to an acute illness that will resolve or due to intoxication from substances) or that they may be more alert later in the day. If the decision can be delayed in these circumstances, it should be.

It becomes more complicated in cases where someone may have the capacity to make decisions about their care and treatment but, due to their mental health, are presenting as a risk to themselves or others and may therefore require a period of treatment as an inpatient. This can either be done *informally*, where the person with capacity consents to an admission to hospital or may be *under section*, if the person meets the criteria for detention under the MHA (1983, 2007) as per the Code of Practice (Department of Health, 2015).

Someone who does not have the capacity to understand and consent to a psychiatric hospital admission should never be informally admitted, even if they are agreeable to admission. They would require either detention under the MHA or under Deprivation of Liberty Safeguards (DOLs) using the MCA. The MHA would be used in a situation where someone's capacity fluctuates or may be regained to ensure appropriate treatment (Department of Health, 2015). Table 6.1 outlines the interaction between capacity and the MHA (Department of Health, 2015). At the time of writing, the Deprivation of Liberty Safeguards (DoLS) under the Mental Capacity Act 2005 remain in force; the Liberty Protection Safeguards created by the Mental Capacity (Amendment) Act 2019 have not yet been implemented.

Understanding the capacity in the context of suicide becomes even more complex. As outlined above, informal admission can be used when

Table 6.1 Interaction between Capacity and the Mental Health Act

	Refusing treatment (whether hospital or declining any treatment for their mental disorder).	Accepting of treatment (whether in hospital or any other treatment for their mental disorder).
Individual has the capacity to consent to treatment.	MHA is the only option available	The MHA is available. Informal admission may also be suitable. DOLs could not be used.
Individual lacks the capacity to consent.	MHA is the only option available	The MHA is available. DOLs may also be available. (See MHA code of practice for England, 13.52, Department of Health, 2015).

someone has the capacity to consent to their care and treatment if they are agreeable to treatment, as this is the least restrictive option. This does not prohibit assessment and detention under the MHA in the future if required (Department of Health, 2015).

However, where it can become challenging is if someone has the capacity to agree to treatment and refuses the recommended treatment. It is important to remember that if a person presents with a clear risk to themselves, due to a diagnosed mental disorder, we have a duty of care to ensure that steps are taken to maintain their safety.

The MCA (or more specifically, stating that a patient "has capacity") has sometimes been misused to withhold treatment from those who ask for support or may be used inappropriately to support a clinical decision not to act on suicidal thoughts when these are reported (Beale, 2022; Beale et al., 2024; Department of Health and Social Care, 2018). Ultimately, this is harmful and telling a patient or service user that they have capacity to make the decision to end their life is likely to increase the risks, while decreasing the trust in health practitioners. People can be left feeling that others do not care about whether they live or die (Aves, 2022). Similarly, professionals have been known to state in an assessment document that a patient is "at risk from death by misadventure". This term has no place in a risk assessment, as "death by misadventure" is a coroner's verdict that describes deaths resulting from voluntary risk-taking that leads to an unintended fatal outcome (Judiciary UK, 2025). Therefore, it is not a recognised medical or psychiatric risk category and does not provide the necessary information required to plan to mitigate the risk. By contrast, documentation that states clearly what the risk is (for example, that a person is at risk from alcohol intoxication and accidental overdose from medication) provides a much clearer picture of the situation and potential avenues for support and intervention

It is important to remember that the hopelessness associated with a person's current mental state is likely to skew their ability to weigh up and understand information, including about potentially effective interventions that are available. For example, if a person is feeling hopeless about the future, they cannot reasonably be expected to believe that they have a chance of recovery. Their current mindset will therefore have an impact on their ability to make informed decisions.

Our priority must be the person's immediate safety, and the state has a responsibility to preserve life if a person is in immediate danger (Keene, 2020). The key is to ask ourselves whether someone has the capacity to consent to the care they need (Beale et al., 2024). Suicide is not a health or care intervention, and so, this is not the decision to assess. While this may change in the future, at the current time, there is no legal framework to support someone to actively take steps to end their life for any reason in the United Kingdom. At the time of writing, assisted dying is not legal in the UK. The Terminally Ill Adults (End of Life) Bill is progressing through Parliament but has not been enacted.

An example in action could be:

1. Imagine Ella attends an appointment where she says that she has suicidal thoughts and is considering taking an overdose. She also mentions having a large collection of tablets but assures you that she has no immediate plan or intent to take them and will be safe when she returns home. Our task is to help Ella understand that keeping the tablets at home increases her risk. We would encourage her to dispose of them appropriately. The question is not whether she has the capacity to decide to overdose, but whether she has the capacity to make decisions about her treatment. In this case, it may involve deciding to keep or dispose of the tablets and accepting additional support if needed. We need to assess whether she understands how having the medication increases the risk of acting on her thoughts impulsively and whether she can weigh up this information. Ella may choose to keep the tablets, which we, as health practitioners, might consider an unwise decision, but it is her right under the MCA. She may share that having the tablets at home feels like a "safety net", while at the same time recognising that having them means she is more likely to overdose in the future.

2. Now, if Ella attends the practice, discloses her suicidal thoughts and medications, and this time expresses an intent to take them as soon as she goes home, our decision-making process would be different. We would need to assess whether Ella has the capacity and willingness to dispose of the medications appropriately to reduce this specific risk and whether she has the capacity to consent to other care and treatment (for example, crisis team intervention or hospitalisation).

    a. If Ella does not have capacity to consent to care and treatment, even if she is agreeable to a hospital admission and it is the appropriate treatment choice, the MHA would be used (see MHA Code of Practice for England, 13.52, Department of Health, 2015).

    b. If Ella has capacity and agrees to admission, she may be admitted as an informal patient for treatment.

115

   c. If Ella has capacity but refuses treatment, to maintain her safety, we must make a clinical decision about the level of risk, which may lead to detention under the MHA.

One of the steps towards understanding the most helpful treatment options is establishing whether a patient is presenting with an acute (sudden onset, usually short in duration, usually moderate to severe) or a chronic (gradual onset or longer duration) problem, as this will determine some elements of our approach.

Understanding a Crisis

A crisis is a short-term highly stressful situation that creates pressure for a quick solution and often leads to a negative outcome (Linehan, 2015). This quick solution to a problem may take the form of suicidal ideas or actions to change emotional and environmental responses.

Thinking specifically about suicide, people can also experience long-term suicidal thoughts without acting upon them. People may find that these chronic thoughts become a strategy for trying to manage emotional pain, and the thoughts may be consistently present or arise in response to specific types of situations (Ronningstam et al., 2024). Patients can experience suicidal thoughts and then also have periods of crisis within this. You can see this in our case study. Ella experienced long-term suicidal and self-harming urges from a very young age. In response to specific situations arising in her life, where her protective factors and risk factors changed, these chronic thoughts escalated and became a crisis in response to those short-term factors.

Tools for Now: Small Changes That Can Make a Big Difference

Managing Professional Anxiety in a High-Risk Situation

Whether thoughts are long term in nature or reaching a crisis, it is likely that our clinical decision-making will be different. However, to work with patients who are experiencing suicidal thoughts, whether acutely or chronically, we must manage our own professional anxiety to make safe clinical decisions that are in the best interests of our patients.

Professional anxiety when working with suicidal patients can present in many ways (Michaud et al., 2023), including:

- Lack of interest or avoidance of the issues
- Anger with the person
- Anxiety and worry
- Feeling overwhelmed and confused
- Feeling rejected by the patient
- Feeling helpless and hopeless

There are several factors that can increase our professional anxiety. These include patients who we are unable to contact or who miss appointments (Dundas et al., 2022; Wolk et al., 2024), and those who are difficult to engage in treatment. Some patients and service users may say one thing to us and another to other professionals (Dundas et al., 2022), leading to a sense of ambiguity about the actual situation. Another aspect that can increase our professional anxiety is having to make a choice, collaboratively or independently, between keeping a patient alive in the short-term and a long-term, more helpful treatment plan. This can feel extremely uncomfortable and risk-laden professionally (Ahmed et al., 2021; Dundas et al., 2022).

An example of this could be if Ella visited the GP, experiencing chronic suicidal ideation and ongoing self-harm, and requests a change in treatment plan. Hearing her distress can increase our anxiety, even though hospitalisation may not be the best option at that time, as she needs to continue her current work with a therapist. We are likely to be left feeling uncomfortable knowing that there is a risk.

Equally uncomfortable is if Ella were to seek help but refuses a hospital admission or a referral to the crisis resolution and home treatment team, when we believe this to be the best treatment option. Requesting her detention under the MHA is likely to place long-term strain on the therapeutic relationship, potentially making her feel unable to seek help from us again. While there is some short-term benefit in keeping her safe, the long-term consequences could impact on her future care and relationships.

Working collaboratively with our patients to formulate treatment plans and to use the skills and techniques that we would teach our patients to manage their emotional responses can help reduce our professional anxiety in these situations (Michaud et al., 2023; Dundas et al., 2022). One technique we can use is to notice our thoughts and modify them, as shown in

Table 6.2 Examples of Anxious Thoughts and Potential Challenges to These

Thought	Challenge examples
"I'm failing my patient".	"I am doing my best in a difficult situation".
"I don't know what to do, I shouldn't be a nurse/health practitioner".	"No nurse or health practitioner will be expert in everything, and professionals ask for help when they need it. It's what makes us better at our jobs".
"What will people think if they find out I can't cope?"	"It's okay to feel uncertain at times. I am trained and capable. Seeking guidance or additional resources is part of providing excellent care".
"Ella always says this, I don't want to hear it again".	"Ella's repeated expressions indicate ongoing distress. By listening empathetically, I can understand her needs and provide meaningful support".

Table 6.2. For example, if we experience thoughts, such as that the situation is hopeless for our patient, or that we don't know what to do, or even that we are incompetent, we need to gently challenge these thoughts within ourselves. It can be helpful to remind ourselves (as we would a patient) that feeling hopeless does not make it a fact that nothing will change, and that we do not have to have all the answers, and that it is expected that we will need additional time and support with complex situations. Changing our thoughts can go a long way towards reducing professional anxiety (Ellis et al., 2018).

Regular reflective practice meetings are recommended to support practitioners to consider their own emotional responses and needs (Royal College of Psychiatrists, 2022). If working in a general hospital, the Psychiatric Liaison Accreditation Network (PLAN) Model of care (Baugh and Talwar, 2022) introduced by the Royal College of Psychiatrists includes supporting reflective practice meetings among acute sector colleagues as a role for the psychiatric liaison team. As part of this model of care, the team will also offer support and advice to colleagues around care of complex patients and situations.

One anxiety-provoking situation is when patients are not receiving appropriate additional treatment. One element that can support our patients to accept treatment from secondary mental health services is more collaborative working as a multidisciplinary team between primary, secondary, and emergency services (Wolk et al., 2024). We can also provide psychoeducation about what to expect once a referral has been made, encourage the person to engage in safety planning, and send them electronic reminders of appointments (Wolk et al., 2024). While these steps may not overcome all barriers, working in more collaborative ways to support treatment plans can increase the likelihood of treatment success and help reduce our professional anxiety.

Working collaboratively with colleagues, managing our own emotions, following our professional guidance, and completing risk assessments will aid us in reducing the worry that may be experienced when working with patients who have suicidal thoughts and intentions. Sharing tools, resources, and information with patients will also help generate feelings of competence and agency.

Supporting Suicidal People – Inspiring Hope

Having the Conversation

There is a common misconception that asking someone about their suicidal thoughts can increase the risk of them acting on those thoughts. However, research has shown that this is not the case (Dazzi et al., 2014). In fact, asking someone directly about suicidal thoughts can provide relief, reduce their sense of isolation, and encourage them to seek help. As explained in Chapter 5, it opens a channel for honest communication and allows the individual to feel heard and supported. When a professional discusses suicidal thoughts with a patient, it is important to approach the topic with sensitivity and care, creating a safe, non-judgemental environment, and using clear, straightforward language. Phrasing such as "I'm concerned about you. Have you been feeling like you want to hurt yourself or end your life?" can be helpful. Avoid asking ambiguous questions like "Have you been feeling like you don't want to be here?" as this could refer to the appointment itself or to a physical or geographical location, rather than to feeling suicidal. Active listening, empathy, and reassurance are key skills that a professional can use to validate the patient's feelings and remind them that they are not alone, offering resources and support to help them through their crisis.

Safety Planning

Creating a safety plan for patients in crisis is a critical step in providing immediate support and preventing self-harm or suicide, and guidance is provided by numerous sources to support this, including the Royal College of Psychiatrists (2018). Professionals should begin by collaboratively developing the plan with the patient, ensuring their active participation and understanding. The safety plan typically includes identifying warning signs that indicate a crisis may be developing, such as changes in mood or behaviour. This can include what might be noticed by the person themselves, but also by others (such as withdrawing or becoming more hostile). Then, it involves identifying and listing coping strategies that the person can use to manage distress, such as deep breathing exercises, engaging in a hobby, or contacting a trusted friend or family member. Remember that advice such as to have a cup of tea or a nice bubble bath can be perceived by patients as belittling their distress and leave them feeling dismissed and invalidated. To be meaningful, they need to identify what the patient finds enjoyable, relaxing, or soothing, and this will be different for everyone. The plan should also include contact information for emergency services, crisis hotlines, and mental health professionals who can provide immediate support.

In addition to these elements, the safety plan should outline a safe environment by discussing removing or securing any potential means of self-harm. This might include things the patient does, such as returning excess medication to the pharmacy to prevent overdose, or things the professional can do, such as modifying prescriptions to be dispensed weekly rather than monthly. Professionals should also work with the patient to identify safe places where they feel comfortable and can go to de-escalate their emotions.

It is essential to regularly review and update safety plans to ensure they remain relevant and effective. The overall goal is to equip and empower the person to take practical steps during a crisis, providing them with a sense of control, which in turn reduces the risk of harm.

Goal Planning

Supporting someone with goal planning during a mental health crisis requires a compassionate and empathic approach. Begin by creating a safe and non-judgemental space where the individual feels heard and understood. Simplify the process by breaking down goals into small, manageable steps. Encourage them to focus on immediate, achievable objectives that can provide a sense of accomplishment. Work together to establish realistic timelines and offer continuous support and reassurance. These goals may focus on immediate safety, such as mitigating any methods they disclose (such as disposing of tablets at the pharmacy) or supporting any plans they have made (for example, avoiding being alone at certain times). Goals could also focus on the causes or triggers for the current presentation, such as seeking therapy for thoughts and feelings, or accessing services that can support them in fulfilling goals around education and employment. Be patient and flexible, understanding that their needs and priorities may shift as they navigate the crisis.

After the Crisis

After a mental health crisis has passed, professionals can work with service users to explore their values and "life worth living goals", as seen in DBT (Linehan, 2015). This process involves helping individuals identify what truly matters to them, such as personal growth, relationships, career aspirations, and overall wellbeing. By aligning therapeutic goals with the person's core values, practitioners can foster a sense of purpose and motivation within patients and service users. This approach supports recovery as well as empowering individuals to build a fulfilling and meaningful life. The collaborative effort between the service user and the therapist ensures that the goals are personalised and achievable, promoting long-term resilience and mental health stability.

Supporting a Person in Crisis: Understanding Specialist Interventions

If someone is experiencing suicidal thoughts and they are unable to keep themselves safe in the here and now, feel hopeless, and are not able to work towards their goals or to bring about changes in their life, there are emergency mental health interventions that may be relevant. As outlined at the start of this chapter, we have a professional duty to initiate appropriate support for the patient. This may be referrals to emergency mental health services such as liaison teams in emergency departments or crisis resolution and home treatment teams. At times, it might be necessary to request an assessment under the MHA to maintain the person's safety.

The least restrictive options should always be used, and it is favourable for crisis services to assess and support the patient in the community where possible. Where this is not safe or practical, admission to a psychiatric hospital may be informal (for an amount of time as agreed in the care plan), or under a Section for a period of assessment (up to 28 days under Section 2 of the MHA) or a longer period of treatment (up to six months under Section 3 of the MHA). Hospitals can be used to help, in the short-term, to preserve safety and support treatment for our patients and reduce our professional anxiety about care. However, it is important to note that the Royal College of Psychiatrists (2020) has highlighted that there is no evidence that hospitalisation reduces the risk of suicide, and that it is not a long-term treatment option. In reality, there is an association between hospitalisation and patients being at higher, rather than lower, risk of suicide (Large et al., 2017). There is little research into the differences between alternative treatment options, partly due to the ethical dilemmas of undertaking this research (Large et al., 2017). A review of records in England found that the risk of suicide for adults was 191 times higher in the three months following discharge as an inpatient from a psychiatric hospital than a similarly matched group (Musgrove et al., 2022). It is challenging to understand all the factors behind why the mental health inpatient wards may place patients at higher risk. It could potentially be that the patients admitted in the first place are at higher risk, hence being admitted, or it could be factors involved in the admission itself that increase the risk (Large and Kapur, 2018), including the ward environment. Without further research, it will be difficult to say.

There are ways that hospitals can support their suicidal patients. This includes people feeling recognised as being suicidal, healthcare professionals seeing the warning signs and having strong therapeutic relationships, alongside the development of individualised care and treatment plans (Berg et al., 2020). This is in line with the advice around use of the MHA to create collaborative care plans.

Another place where patients are likely to present in a crisis is the emergency department, whether prior to a suicide attempt or following a suicide attempt. Mental health liaison services are available in hospitals, both to support wards within the general hospital and the emergency departments. These multidisciplinary teams work with colleagues based in the acute setting to provide assessments and treatments to patients presenting with a mental health crisis, and to offer support to colleagues who are not trained in mental health.

The PLAN model was introduced and established in 2009 by the Royal College of Psychiatrists in an effort to improve both the quality of liaison services and the sustainability of these services (Baugh and Talwar, 2022). The standards outline expected staffing levels and interventions available, to include assessments, therapy, follow-up sessions, and advice around medication prescribing with specialists.

Once a referral has been made, if this is an emergency, the patient should be seen within an hour of the referral. If not an emergency but a request for support with someone's mental health, this must happen within 24 hours (Baugh and Talwar, 2022). Assessments should be a full psychosocial assessment, and an emergency mental health care plan should be created and put in place. The outcomes of the assessment will vary and may include a scheduled follow-up of someone's care, discharge if the crisis has been resolved, referral to secondary mental health services in the community, talking therapy services, or potentially requesting a MHA assessment where this is the recommended course of action.

Finally, there are numerous third sector organisations, such as the Samaritans, that also offer support to people when they are experiencing a suicidal crisis. Some people make frequent use of these services, often as part of a wider support network and alongside other services (Coveney et al., 2012). Coveney et al. (2012) found that people who had contacted the Samaritans felt more positive following the call and that the people they surveyed attributed this to feeling listened to and understood and, perhaps most importantly, having found alternative solutions to their problems. Useful contact numbers and further information on availability for UK Helplines can be found in Table 6.3 below.

Table 6.3 Sources of Support in a Crisis *(Correct at the Time of Publication)*

UK helpline numbers		
Mind	0300 102 1234	9 am – 6 pm, Monday – Friday
Samaritans	116 123	24 hours a day 365 days a year
SANEline	0300 304 7000	4:30 pm – 10:00 pm daily
National suicide prevention helpline	0800 689 5652	6 pm – midnight daily
SHOUT	Text SHOUT to: 85258	24/7 text service
NHS	111 Option 2	24 hours a day, 365 days a year

Summary of Learning Points

This chapter has explored a wide range of approaches to supporting practitioners, as they help people find hope during a suicidal crisis:

- The Mental Health Act and Deprivation of Liberty Safeguards under the Mental Capacity Act have been identified as potentially being used to detain someone for their safety if they are experiencing a crisis.
- It has been explained that capacity cannot be used in a statement whereby an individual is deemed to have "capacity to act on suicidal thoughts" or as a reason for professionals to refuse to offer treatment.
- Professional anxieties around managing risk have been acknowledged as real and understandable. Various tools and techniques can be used to support us with this, such as thought modification, which can help in managing our emotional responses to the challenges arising when working with a suicidal patient.
- It has been emphasised that it is important to have conversations about suicide and to support people to plan for their own safety when they are experiencing suicidal thoughts and urges.
- There are specialist crisis services available, and hospitalisation is an option if it is required to maintain immediate safety, although risks associated with hospital admission have also been identified.
- In the long term, after the crisis has passed, it is important to support people to work on identifying why their life is worth living.

Questions for Reflection and Discussion

1. How can you and your colleagues promote the use of more constructive, collaborative, and validating approaches to equipping and empowering people you work with who may be experiencing suicidal thoughts and intentions?

2. Identify any times when capacity statements have been used to support your decision-making in practice. Were any of these statements about capacity erroneously applied?

3. What changes can you and your colleagues make going forward in considering the interactions between the MHA, MCA, and capacity for decision-making?

4. Identify ways in which you or colleagues may sometimes act in risk-avoidant ways due to anxieties around suicidal thoughts and actions among the patients and service users with whom you work.

5. In what ways do you currently manage your professional anxiety when working with high-risk patients? Are there any more helpful ways you could find to manage this?

Recommended Follow-up Reading

Beale, C., Lee-Davey, J., Lee, T. and Keene, A.R. (2024). Mental capacity in practice part 2: Capacity and the suicidal patient. *BJPsych Advances*. 30(1): 11–20.

Hallett, N. (2024). Assessing mental capacity: Tensions, values and duties. *BJPsych Advances*. 30(1): 21–23.

Jamison, J.M., Brady, M., Fang, A., Bùi, T.M.N., Wolk, C.B., Davis, M., Beidas, R.S., Young, J.F., Mautone, J.A., Jager-Hyman, S. and Becker-Haimes, E.M. (2025). A qualitative examination of clinician anxiety about suicide prevention and its impact on clinical practice. *Community Mental Health Journal*. 61(3): 568–575.

Mental Capacity, Law and Policy (2022). Suicide and the (mis)use of capacity – in conversation with Dr Chloe Beale. Available online at: https://www.mentalcapacitylawandpolicy.org.uk/suicide-and-the-misuse-of-capacity-in-conversation-with-dr-chloe-beale/ - A video about capacity and use of MHA

Richardson, G. (2013). Mental capacity in the shadow of suicide: What can the law do? *International Journal of Law in Context*. 9(1): 87–105.

References

Ahmed, N., Barlow, S., Reynolds, L., Drey, N., Begum, F., Tuudah, E. and Simpson, A. (2021). Mental health professionals' perceived barriers and enablers to shared decision making in risk assessment and risk management: A qualitative systematic review. *BMC Psychiatry*. 21: 594.

Aves, W. (2022). "If you are not a patient they like, then you have capacity." *Exploring Mental Health Patient and Survivor Experiences of being told "You have the Capacity to End Your Life". Psychiatry is Driving Me Mad*. Available online at: https://www.psychiatryisdrivingmemad.co.uk/post/if-you-are-not-a-patient-they-like-then-you-have-capacity. [Accessed 15th August 2025].

Barnett, P., Tickell, A., Osborn, T., Delamain, H., Fonagy, P., Pilling, S. and Gibbon, L. (2024). Help-seeking and disclosure in university students with suicidal thoughts and self-harm: A systematic review. *International Journal of Mental Health and Addiction*. 2024: 1–78.

Baugh, C. and Talwar, K. (eds.) (2022). PLAN: 7th edition standards. *Royal College of Psychiatrists*. Available online at: https://www.rcpsych.ac.uk/docs/default-source/

improving-care/ccqi/quality-networks/psychiatric-liaison-services-plan/
plan---7th-edition-standards.pdf?sfvrsn=b1a9b1a3_3. [Accessed 17th January 2025].

Beale, C. (2022). Magical thinking and moral injury: Exclusion culture in psychiatry. *BJPsych Bulletin*. 46: 16–19.

Beale, C., Lee-Davey, J., Lee, T. and Keene, A.R. (2024). Mental capacity in practice part 2: Capacity and the suicidal patient. *BJPsych Advances*. 30: 11–20.

Berg, S.H., Rørtveit, K., Walby, F.A. and Aase, K. (2020). Safe clinical practice for patients hospitalised in mental health wards during a suicidal crisis: Qualitative study of patient experiences. *BMJ Open*. 10: e040088.

Coveney, C.M., Pollock, K., Armstrong, S. and Moore, J. (2012). Callers' experiences of contacting a national suicide prevention helpline. *Crisis: The Journal of Crisis Intervention and Suicide Prevention*. 33(6): 313–324.

Dazzi, T., Gribble, R., Wessely, S. and Fear, N.T. (2014). Does asking about suicide and related behaviours induce suicidal ideation? What is the evidence? *Psychological Medicine*. 44(16): 3361–3363.

Department of Health (2005). *Mental Capacity Act*. London: HMSO.

Department of Health (2015). Mental Health Act 1983: Code of practice (updated 2015). London: HMSO. Available online at: https://assets.publishing.service.gov.uk/media/5a80a774e5274a2e87dbb0f0/MHA_Code_of_Practice.PDF. [Accessed 15th August 2025].

Department of Health and Social Care (2018). Modernising the Mental Health Act. Increasing Choice, Reducing Compulsion. Available online at: https://assets.publishing.service.gov.uk/media/5c6596a7ed915d045f37798c/Modernising_the_Mental_Health_Act_-_increasing_choice__reducing_compulsion.pdf. [Accessed 24th January 2025].

Dundas, I., Hjeltnes, A., Schanche, E. and Stige, S.H. (2022). Does it get easier over time? Psychologists' experiences of working with suicidal patients. *Death Studies*. 46(2): 458–466.

Ellis, T.E., Schwartz, J.A.J. and Rufino, K.A. (2018). Negative reactions of therapists working with suicidal patients: A CBT/mindfulness perspective on "countertransference". *Journal of Cognitive Therapy*. 11: 80–99.

Gibbons, R. (2024). Someone is to blame: The impact of suicide on the mind of the bereaved (including clinicians). *BJPsych Bulletin*. 49(1): 36–40.

Hawton, K., Lascelles, K., Pitman, A., Gilbert, S. and Silverman, M. (2022). Assessment of suicide risk in mental health practice: Shifting from prediction to therapeutic assessment, formulation, and risk management. *Lancet Psychiatry*. 9: 922–928.

Healthcare Quality Improvement Partnership (2025). Suicide and safety in mental health (NCISH). Available online at: https://www.hqip.org.uk/resource/mental-health-ncish-feb25/?form=MG0AV3. [Accessed 15th February 2025].

Judiciary UK (2025). Courts and tribunals judiciary. *Chapter 15: Conclusions*. Available online at: https://www.judiciary.uk/guidance-and-resources/conclusions/. [Accessed 15th August 2025].

Keene, R.K. (2020). Mental capacity law and policy: *Capacity and Suicide*. Available online at: https://www.mentalcapacitylawandpolicy.org.uk/capacity-and-suicide/. [Accessed 15th February 2025].

Large, M.M., Chung, D.T., Davidson, M., Weiser, M. and Ryan, C.J. (2017). In-patient suicide: Selection of people at risk, failure of protection and the possibility of causation. *BJPsych Open*. 3(3): 102–105.

Large, M.M. and Kapur, N. (2018). Psychiatric hospitalisation and the risk of suicide. *The British Journal of Psychiatry*. 212: 269–273.

Linehan, M. (2015). *DBT Skills Training Manual*. (2nd ed). New York: The Guildford Press.

Michaud, L., Greenway, K.T., Corbeil, S., Bourquin, C. and Richard-Devantoy, S. (2023). Countertransference towards suicidal patients: A systematic review. *Current Psychology*. 42: 416–430.

Millard, C. (2015). *A History of Self-Harm in Britain. A Genealogy of Cutting and Overdosing*. Basingstoke: Palgrave Macmillan.

Musgrove, R., Carr, M.J., Kapur, N., Chew-Graham, C.A., Mughal, F., Ashcroft, D.M. and Webb, R.T. (2022). Suicide and other causes of death among working-age and older adults in the year after discharge from in-patient mental healthcare in England: Matched cohort study. *The British Journal of Psychiatry*. 221: 468–475.

Office for Health Improvement and Disparities (2025). Statistical report: near to real-time suspected suicide surveillance (nRTSSS) for England for the 15 months to October 2024. Available online at: https://www.gov.uk/government/statistics/near-to-real-time-suspected-suicide-surveillance-nrtsss-for-england/statistical-report-near-to-real-time-suspected-suicide-surveillance-nrtsss-for-england-for-the-15-months-to-august-2023?form=MG0AV3. [Accessed 15th August 2025].

Office for National Statistics (2024). Suicides in England and Wales: 2023 registrations. Available online at: https://www.ons.gov.uk/peoplepopulationandcommunity/birthsdeathsandmarriages/deaths/bulletins/suicidesintheunitedkingdom/2023. [Accessed 15th August 2025].

Oxford University Press (2024). Oxford learner's dictionaries: Commit (verb). Available online at: https://www.oxfordlearnersdictionaries.com/definition/english/commit?q=commit. [Accessed 15th August 2025].

Ronningstam, E., Schechter, M., Herbstman, B. and Goldbalatt, N. (2024). Chronic suicidal ideations: A risk or a protection. *Research in Psychotherapy: Psychopathology, Process and Outcome*. 27: 764.

Royal College of Psychiatrists (2018). Safety planning guidance. Available online at: ohft-safety-planning-guidance.pdf. [Accessed 15th August 2025].

Royal College of Psychiatrists (2020) Self-harm and suicide in adults: Final report of the Patient Safety Group. Available online at: https://www.rcpsych.ac.uk/docs/default-source/improving-care/better-mh-policy/college-reports/college-report-cr229-self-harm-and-suicide.pdf?sfvrsn=b6fdf395_10. [Accessed 15th August 2025].

Royal College of Psychiatrists (2022). Report CR234: Supporting mental health staff following the death of a patient by suicide: A prevention and postvention framework. Available online at: https://www.rcpsych.ac.uk/docs/default-source/improving-care/better-mh-policy/college-reports/college-report-cr234-staff-support-following-patient-suicide.pdf?sfvrsn=f6571a69_12. [Accessed 15th August 2025].

Wolk, C.B., Pieri, M., Weiss, S.E., Harrison, J., Khazanov, G.K., Candon, M., Oslin, D.W., Press, M.J., Anderson, E., Famiglio, E., Buttenheim, A. and Jager-Hyman, S. (2024). Engaging primary care patients at risk for suicide in mental health treatment: User insights to inform implementation strategy design. *BMC Primary Care.* 25: 371.

7

Bereavement Support Following a Death by Suicide

John Whitebrook

Case Study

Roy's Story

I will never forget the Monday morning that my older son called me at 8 am. As soon as I saw his number, I had a sense of foreboding. I recall him saying his younger brother "is gone" together with an immediate understanding of what that meant, countered by an overwhelming sense of denial and panic. The rest of that day, and the following months, are a blur of events and emotions, punctuated with moments of clarity. I was in a constant daze and unsure of everything, with no confidence in my ability to function normally in any capacity. Much of the time, it felt like I was an observer, watching myself go through the motions of daily life. One thing I became single-minded about was delivering a eulogy and I spent a lot of time thinking about what I wanted to cover. The delivery of it went well, which was (and still is) extremely important to me.

In terms of anything practical, I was useless and relied heavily on others, especially my wife. I thought of my son in every waking moment and his loss totally dominated my day-to-day life, month after month after month. At night, I couldn't get to sleep, with images flashing through my mind, and I'd lie awake for hours. Eventually, I did sleep but then didn't want to leave my bed the next day, and spent many hours huddled under the covers. I was later diagnosed with clinical depression.

I did go back to work, after a few weeks, but was a shadow of my former self and very much went through the motions. Luckily, I was

DOI: 10.4324/9781003635611-8

in a senior position and could largely get by for a while, but my confidence and ability to lead had evaporated. Being put in pressurised situations found me out and I struggled to cope.

I started therapy soon after my son's death and also started attending the peer support group meetings run by Survivors of Bereavement by Suicide (SoBS). The former was initially beneficial in helping me align my thoughts, and the latter invaluable in that it put me in contact with others who welcomed me and really "got it". Many times, since then, in group sessions, we've talked about being members of a club no one ever wants to join but, once you're in it, you feel a sense of camaraderie and kinship impossible to find elsewhere.

I'm lucky in that the loss brought my family together, whereas, as I've learnt from the sharing of others, suicide is more often divisive. After a year of being on autopilot, on the first anniversary of my son's death, the mental dam I'd unwittingly built broke, and a tsunami of emotions swept through me. A family intervention had me at my GP soon after. She was (and still is) massively empathetic and supportive. I was prescribed medication (which I was on and off for a while – now off) but also strongly urged to maintain the therapy and peer support. After a few more months, and pressure being piled on, I had to take time of work – that was extended and extended until I ended up retiring early. The loss of career and status was another blow.

After a period of stability, I became a volunteer meeting facilitator with SoBS and helping others has significantly helped me. In parallel, I went through several therapists, including one where I did CBT and was clinically diagnosed with PTSD, but although I made progress, I still felt stuck. A few years in, my wife suggested EMDR and that helped me make a massive breakthrough, in terms of processing some specific memories and associated guilt. In conjunction, listening and talking to others in the SoBS sessions, facilitated an epiphany that, although I had personally contributed to the whole of my son's life, other factors influenced who he was, and ultimately, he made the decision to end his life for reasons of his own. I know I'll miss him always and the guilt will continually be there, but the gut-wrenching ache has largely abated, and I have accepted that I can live a meaningful life whilst cherishing his memory.

Introduction

The global suicide rate is around 760,000 per year, of whom 70% are male (Ilic and Ilic, 2022). It has been estimated that 135 people are exposed to each suicide because they knew the person (Cerel et al., 2019). Studies suggest that over their lifespan, more than a third of people experience medium to severe emotional trauma related to losing someone to suicide (Sandford et al., 2021). Survey data suggest approximately 60 people are deeply affected by each suicide, and annual exposure to suicides has been estimated to involve between 48 and 500 million people (Pitman et al., 2014). The term "suicide-loss survivor(s)" (SLS) is utilised in this chapter and refers to those who have experienced the suicide of a close family member or a friend and face persistent, distressing trauma (Levi-Belz and Birnbaum, 2022). The term differentiates those who survive a suicide attempt.

Chapter Aims

This chapter focuses on understanding, and thereby better supporting, the life-changing experience of becoming an SLS, and includes:

- The impact of losing someone to suicide.
- Stigma associated with, and myths relating to, suicide loss.
- Prolonged grief disorder (PGD) and post-traumatic growth (PTG).
- Support available to SLS.

Suicide and Bereavement

The care for those bereaved by suicide is designated "postvention" and is also recognised as a key suicide prevention measure for SLS (Jordan, 2017). Exposure to suicide loss and attempts has been related to greater suicidal behaviour (Hill et al., 2020) and has been found to increase the risk of suicide by 65% in young adults (Pitman et al., 2016). Cognitively, some SLS may find the loss of a loved one makes the concept of suicide more acceptable, but others may reject this notion, while some encounter conflicting perceptions (Jones et al., 2024).

Reporting of celebrity suicides often leads to a cluster of suicides (risk increase of 13%), especially where the method is divulged (risk increase of 30%) (Niederkrotenthaler et al., 2020). There are a variety of ways in which suicidality may be transmitted, including traditional means such as news and entertainment, as well as via social media, plus there can be suicide clusters in specific locations (Pirkis et al., 2024). Clusters are more common in young people, as opposed to adults (Hawton et al., 2020) and are sometimes associated with specific geographic locations, which, due to their notoriety, attract those with suicidal ideation. Restricting access to such locations, and to means in general, has been found to be effective in reducing suicides (Schlichthorst et al., 2022).

Social media has been found to act as a means of contagion, in relation to suicide clusters (known as the "Werther effect"), but it can also be protective (this is known as the "Papageno effect") (Calvo et al., 2024). There are many studies suggesting that a variety of socio-economic factors influence suicide risk, but the complexity and interactions between factors confound attempts at prediction overall (Huang et al., 2017). Higher suicide rates have been noted for healthcare professionals, including physicians, veterinarians, and nurses (Dalum et al., 2024).

The Impact of Losing Someone to Suicide

SLS very often perceive that their lives are falling apart, that they have been irrevocably changed by their loss, and experience huge guilt, combined with frustration relating to most, if not all, of the institutions they have inter-actions with, both pre- and post-loss. Many SLS internalise their angst and stress, presenting an outward appearance of coping when, in fact, they are silently in agony (Whitebrook and Churchyard, 2025). The search for answers, guilt, stigma, isolation, and suicidal ideation tend to differentiate SLS from other types of mourner and undermines their certainty in the safety of others they care for and their ability to protect them (Jordan, 2020).

A rise in the risk of major depression, anxiety, post-traumatic stress disor-der (PTSD), which is often under-diagnosed (Sanford et al., 2016), and PGD, with these often co-occurring, has been associated with suicide bereave-ment (Grafiadeli et al., 2022). Suicide bereavement involves complex, inter-related factors that affect how survivors adapt and cope, both immediately after their loss and for years as they seek meaning in their experience. Any service providing support to SLS should consider the wider impacts of what has occurred, and how their assistance fits within the overall framework of suicide bereavement. Postvention may be considered within the framework of a comprehensive Suicide Bereavement Model (Whitebrook et al., 2025), which provides insight into the scope of suicide bereavement and exemplifies the interrelationships among various support components.

Self-Management When Interacting with SLS

Those impacted by suicides include healthcare practitioners, ranging from those that interacted with the individual lost, first responders, and those that interact with the SLS. Losing a service user to suicide can be deleterious to healthcare practitioners' mental health, undermine their confidence, and lead to them questioning the adequacy of their training and support, with these feelings often being more common amongst female and older practitioners (Murphy et al., 2019; Sandford et al., 2021). Paramedics can find their work environment lacking in empathy and support despite frequently attending suicides, which are sometimes of colleagues, due to the high suicide rate in the profession (Nelson et al., 2020; Witczak-Błoszyk et al., 2022). Healthcare practitioners who encounter SLS, having not been involved prior to the loss, can still be affected by the suffering they witness in others. Being affected by patients' ordeals can lead to secondary traumatic stress, vicarious traumatisation, and compassion fatigue (Hansel and Saltzman, 2024).

Managing Your Thoughts and Feelings When a Service User Dies by Suicide

The loss of a service user to suicide results in sadness and often concern, along with a level of self-recrimination (Gibbons et al., 2019). Training and preparation for the possibility of losing a service user to suicide can be highly beneficial in helping you cope. Such training should encompass the impact of becoming an SLS and the support that is available to you (Sandford et al., 2021). In addition to embracing this preparedness, it is important that you do not try to deal with the situation in isolation but seek support from a senior figure (including a debrief on the incident), as well as peers. Reflect on practices relating to the loss, understand any procedural corollaries, and speak with those who are in a position to liaise with family members of the deceased. Connection with the latter should be on a level which is emotionally meaningful, being aware of their needs, as well as the support available to them (Gibbons et al., 2019).

Stress and self-doubt, arising from the loss, may lead you to be over-cautious with other patients and service users, including additional consultations with colleagues, and increased hospitalisations (Erbuto et al., 2021). Masking your feelings and distress or not receiving adequate support can be detrimental in the long term (Gutin, 2019b). However, the experience of dealing with the loss of a patient or service user to suicide can provide you with enhanced skills to deal with any future losses of this type (Murphy et al., 2019) as well as facilitate your professional development (Gutin, 2019a). Being aware of the risk that you may encounter secondary traumatic stress, together with acknowledging potential impacts related to this on yourself (for example, understanding your own strengths and weaknesses), can help mitigate the effects, as can seeking help, such as counselling or engaging with a community of practice (Bride et al., 2024; Murphy et al., 2019). Organised and facilitated, formal peer support groups could also be beneficial to you when coming to terms with the suicide of a service user or patient (Tamworth et al., 2022).

Throughout, it is key that you recognise that your feelings and reactions are unique to you, as an individual, and that your needs may be different to those of others (Causer et al., 2019).

Managing Your Thoughts and Feelings When a Colleague Dies by Suicide

In the event of a colleague's suicide, you will be the SLS, and it is important that you engage in the approaches outlined here, for service users and patients, as the experience of interacting with other SLS in no way confers you with immunity from the impact of suicide bereavement. You will need the accessible and sustained support of others within your organisation to navigate through this very difficult time. If you find yourself in the role of supporter, it is vital that you too are supported (Spiers et al., 2024). The most common emotions you are likely to experience, subsequent to a colleague's suicide, are shock and anger, the latter of which can lead to anxiety, embarrassment and uncertainty (Causer et al., 2022).

Not all the services and support you would ideally want and need to access may exist or be available at any point in time. From an organisational perspective, you may feel pressure to conduct "business as usual". Even if this is the case, it is important that you have the opportunity to talk to colleagues and to take the time needed to process the loss (Causer et al., 2025).

Stigma Associated with, and Myths Relating to, Suicide Loss

Suicide remains highly stigmatised, often exacerbating shame and leading to social estrangement (Goulah-Pabst, 2023). SLS often find others to be judgemental, with a tendency for them to avoid the topic. This contributes to the withdrawal and potential amplification of anguish for the SLS (Evans and Abrahamson, 2020). Blame can be internalised and, while SLS can band together for support, a suicide loss can also be divisive, causing rifts within, and between, family and friends (Peters et al., 2016b). SLS very often have a shift in priorities and can lose interest in aspects of life about which they were previously enthusiastic, which can lead to them inherently self-isolating (Whitebrook and Churchyard, 2025). Institutional lack of understanding, or insensitivity, regarding the needs of SLS including by healthcare practitioners, can intensify, rather than alleviate, SLS emotional trauma (Peters et al., 2016a).

Common misconceptions (Gibbons, 2023) regarding suicide pervade society, and suicide myths can also be inherent in the perspectives of some healthcare practitioners (Ayala Romera et al., 2024; Bahamón et al., 2024). Tabloid newspapers have been found to disseminate typical suicide fallacies, hampering public awareness of the realities and perpetuating stigma around suicide (Till et al., 2018). Belief in suicide myths may be correlated with age as well as ethnicity (Nicholas et al., 2020).

In addition to the academic papers noted above, there are many sources listing commonly held suicide-related myths, which can be easily found using a web search.

PGD and PTG

Acute grief most often transitions to integrated grief, as SLS adapt to their changed existence over time. However, for some people, the dire pain and suffering related to their bereavement perpetuates and has been described as complicated grief (Levi-Belz and Lev-Ari, 2019a). More recently, the term PGD has been included in the 5th edition of the Diagnostic and Statistical Manual of Mental Disorders (DSM-5-TR) and the International Classification of Diseases 11th Revision (ICD-11) (Lenferink et al., 2021, 2022). A subgroup of SLS become fixated on those they have lost, along with persistence

135

of their emotional suffering and maladjusted behaviours (Levi-Belz and Ben-Yaish, 2022). In dealing with SLS it is important that you look out for the signs of PGD and that you are aware that those afflicted will require additional, and more protracted, support to adjust to their losses (Grafiadeli et al., 2022).

Conversely, after the initial shock and distress begin to abate, some SLS will adapt to their situation and use their adverse experience as an opportunity for a positive change in the way they view the world. Demonstration of such PTG is often mediated by the extent to which they share their feelings, receive support socially, and how they relate to others (Levi-Belz and Lev-Ari, 2019b; Levi-Belz et al., 2021). Additional predictors for PTG that have been identified include time since bereavement, gender, whether an SLS has lost one or more loved ones, their individual grieving process (Creegan et al., 2025), and their level of self-forgiveness (Gilo et al., 2022).

It is important to be aware that SLS' healing is not a linear process but cyclical in nature, reflecting their own ruminations (Morrissey et al., 2024) or how they are treated (Marek and Oexle, 2024). Relapses may be triggered by anything that brings the death of their loved one to mind (Jordan, 2020), which can include hearing other people relating their losses (Kaspersen et al., 2022; Morrissey et al., 2024) and dealing with the procedural consequences, such as an inquest (Spillane et al., 2019).

Support Available to SLS

Most SLS especially in the initial period post-bereavement, struggle with trying to make sense of why their loved one took their own life, including why the relationship they had together was not enough for them to want to live. They continually ask themselves questions such as whether they, or others, could have averted the suicide, and whether anyone was responsible. These perpetual dilemmas do not have simple answers, or possibly any answers at all, and can be barriers to comprehending their real needs (Jordan, 2020).

A major alleviant of SLS suffering can be simple acts of kindness (Peters et al., 2016a). Healthcare practitioners can be enormously helpful to SLS by sign-posting assistance available outside of the healthcare system (Jordan, 2020), including organisations specific to the SLS' locality (Bell et al., 2024). Uptake of any support offered to SLS will be influenced by a multitude of factors in addition to their state of mind at the time. Religiosity is a factor, with some SLS embracing spirituality, while others eschew it (Čepulienė and Skruibis, 2022). Similarly, with ethnicity, some cultures tend to directly impugn SLS (Ali and Rehna, 2023) or even ostracise them (Ohayi, 2019). There are conflicting views on whether pathologising grief is detrimental to the care of patients (Prigerson et al., 2024) and is something you should consider when dealing with SLSs. The main drivers, regarding patient receptivity to postvention, include their underlying attitude towards professional psychological care, rather than the specifics of their loss and grief, and the accessibility and continuity of care. The latter covers timeliness, location, duration, perceived competence (of healthcare practitioners), finances, and lack of information (Geleželytė et al., 2020).

Across all the types of support available to SLS, it is important to be mindful that they are a cohort vulnerable to suicide and that "postvention is prevention" (Jordan, 2017).

Support from the Healthcare System

Many SLS consult their primary care provider, regarding their mental health, and may engage with them over a long period. Despite similar levels of need, most of these contacts are with female SLS, rather than males, and bereaved siblings are also less likely to seek such help (Bélanger et al., 2024). Primary care providers view bereavement support to be part of their roles but often consider themselves lacking in training and resources needed to be effective, which both diminishes their confidence and is especially an issue for patients suffering with prolonged grief, with clinicians also often lacking up-to-date awareness of grief models (Pearce et al., 2021).

SLS struggle with the wherewithal to locate assistance, especially in the immediate aftermath of their loss, and so a proactive outreach programme would be beneficial, but the infrastructure for this is missing (Kaspersen et al., 2022). SLS often face complex relationships with healthcare organisations, which can be adversarial, where they feel those lost were not sufficiently cared for, or that the family was excluded and thereby not able to intervene appropriately. These aspects can lead to a lack of engagement with healthcare systems post-bereavement (Kaspersen et al., 2022; Whitebrook and Churchyard, 2025).

While primary care providers are well-placed to assist (Suija et al., 2022), they often lack sufficient awareness to guide SLS on the relevant services that are available, including voluntary organisations (Foggin et al., 2016;

Nic an Fhailí et al., 2016). Holistically, there is a lack of a clear picture on SLS help-seeking behaviour, service coordination and hand-offs, traceability of care, and overall outcomes (Kaspersen et al., 2022), and many patients are fearful of a medication-only based approach (Nic an Fhailí et al., 2016).

These complexities highlight that you will require a complete knowledge of the services available nationally, as well as in your local area, and be sufficiently trained or able to access support from those more experienced to deal with the manifold needs of SLS.

Peer Support Groups

Peer support groups stand out, in that they provide SLS with a means to interact with their fellow suicide-bereaved, providing them with a unique sense that others understand what they are going through (Peters et al., 2016a), that they are not alone in their struggles (O'Connell et al., 2023), and that they can openly discuss their grief in a safe space (Morrissey et al., 2024). Rigorous and standardised evaluation of peer support is limited (Abbate et al., 2024), although a systematic review highlighted that SLS perceive significant benefit from peer support group attendance, including meaning-making, but noted that consistency and volunteer facilitator capabilities are key factors in promoting optimal effects (Adshead et al., 2025). The effectiveness of peer support can also be limited by the immotive nature of sharing and the behaviours of other SLSs (Kaspersen et al., 2022).

In the wake of their bereavement, SLS may be unaware of the peer support available and how to engage with organisations that provide it, so you should be ready to signpost them to the relevant national and local providers, bearing in mind that such support may be the most immediately available.

Support from Other Sources

Some charities provide telephone support lines, email support, and online forums as adjuncts to peer support group meetings. Research has suggested that online resources (for example, forums, social media, and memorial websites) may be beneficial, but more evaluative work needs to be done to verify positive outcomes (Lestienne et al., 2021). Publicly sharing the experiences of their loss can also be beneficial to SLS (Kirchner and Niederkrotenthaler, 2024).

Awareness of all the options available and consideration of the right time for SLS to engage with each of them are invaluable in providing SLSs with opportunities to maximise their potential for dealing with their loss.

Tools for Now: Small Changes That Can Make a Big Difference

There is no "one-size-fits-all" approach to supporting SLS, due to variations in relationships, attachment to those lost, situation, and timeframe, so you should bear in mind some key aspects of SLS' support needs:

- Simple acts of kindness, understanding, and empathy can make a significant difference to SLS.
- SLS are very often bewildered and confused, and so need help navigating the support services available to them.
- SLS receptivity to support can be modulated by numerous factors including culture, religion, gender, attitude towards the healthcare system, and labelling them as having a condition.
- PTSD is under-diagnosed in people experiencing suicide loss and so you should be mindful of potential indicators of this.
- SLS needs vary over time but may be constrained by the services available to them, for example, in the first few months, post-bereavement, psychotherapy may not be an option (due to waiting list and/or moratorium), but peer support will likely be immediately available (with a caveat that while often providing great comfort, it can be emotionally triggering).
- Awareness of the emotional impact of dealing with SLS (or you own loss) is paramount with respect to both self-care and your interactions with those you support.

SLS very often rely on suicide loss-specific bereavement support provided by charities, which include:

- Australia: Lifeline Australia – https://www.lifeline.org.au/get-help/information-and-support/bereaved-by-suicide/
- Ireland: Healing Untold Grief Groups (HUGG) – https://hugg.ie/

- UK: Survivors of Bereavement by Suicide (SoBS) – https://uksobs.com/
- US: Alliance of Hope for Suicide Loss Survivors – https://allianceofhope.org/

Longer-Term Approaches: Therapies in Suicide Loss

Studies have shown that many SLS seek therapy and that their needs for this are generally greater than for those bereaved by other means. Perceived stigma is not necessarily a barrier to seeking professional help, and therapy can help reduce grief-related indicators (Geležėlytė et al., 2020). Specifically, therapy focused on helping SLS process interpersonal aspects, so that they can reassimilate with family and social networks, may be vital in mitigating depression associated with suicide loss (Levi-Belz and Birnbaum, 2022; Levi-Belz and Ben-Yaish, 2022), along with helping the person to contextualise their loss and to be able to reinvest in their life moving forward (Jordan, 2020).

Feedback from SLS suggests a favourable perception of therapy, although professionals may often miss the signs and symptoms of PTSD, commonly experienced by SLS, suggesting more training may be beneficial regarding that aspect and the specifics of suicide loss/trauma (Sanford et al., 2016).

Cognitive Behavioural Therapy (CBT) has been shown to be effective in helping SLS deal with their grief (Romero-Moreno et al., 2024) and online CBT may be effective in alleviating aspects of SLS grief in some groups (Treml et al., 2021; Wagner et al., 2022). Eye Movement Desensitisation and Reprocessing (EMDR) has also proven viable for assisting those with prolonged grief, where grieving process blocks have been well-defined (Spicer, 2024), specifically for SLS (Jordan, 2020).

Timeliness is a factor, with provision of therapy within three months of the bereavement proving more valuable than if delivered later. SLS proactivity, in seeking help, may account somewhat for this, but it also suggests that more immediate therapeutic intervention is optimal (Sanford et al., 2016)

Healthcare organisational procedures and/or insurance limitations may promote delayed and/or time-limited therapy, so it is important that you are aware of any constraints regarding therapies that can be offered and delivered. Ideally, you should look to match SLS with therapists who have the appropriate skillset and experience, to maximise the potential for benefit, and maintain contact with SLS to verify progress.

Summary of Learning Points

This chapter has explored the following theoretical and practical approaches to understanding and supporting people living as SLS:

- Suicide bereavement is highly complex and has many facets:
  - Mental health problems including, anxiety, depression, PTSD, and PGD.
  - Physical health problems may manifest related to trauma.
  - Social issues may arise from blame, stigma, and family or cultural divisiveness.
  - SLS may be re-traumatised by factors such as the inquest process, dealing with the deceased's estate, work stress, and loss of a sense of self-determination.
- Losing someone to suicide can fundamentally and irrevocably change SLS' lives.
- Suicide bereavement is different to that arising from deaths by other means.
- Suicide bereavement can have long-term negative effects on SLS' health, and they are a high-risk group for suicide.
- Being an SLS can be highly stigmatising, which can result in isolation and compound the effects of trauma.
- Numerous ways exist to assist SLS (medication, talking therapy, CBT, EMDR, and peer support), which are most effectively used in combination and tailored to individual needs, over time.
- In terms of healthcare and other support for SLS:
  - Therapy options should be specific to the needs of SLS and may change over time.
  - Third sector support options may vary based on locality.
  - It is important to constantly glean feedback, to hone approaches, and to tailor solutions to individual needs where practicable.

Questions for Reflection and Discussion

1. Are you fully aware of the depth and breadth of the impact of losing someone you care for to suicide?

2. Do you feel sufficiently prepared to deal with someone that has lost a loved one to suicide? Training is very important along with consulting with colleagues who have relevant experience. Prior dealings with SLS will facilitate honing of your approach.

3. Are you aware of all the options available for healthcare support for SLS and what has been found to be most effective?

4. What recommendations would you make to a SLS to manage their grief? Are you familiar with steps that could facilitate post-traumatic growth?

5. What barriers may arise for you personally when working with people who have been bereaved by suicide? Are there situations or needs that you have that it is important to be aware of so that you can better support others?

Recommended Follow-Up Reading

Andriessen, K., Krysinska, K. and Grad, O.T. (2017). *Postvention in Action: The International Handbook of Suicide Bereavement Support*. Newburyport, MA: Hogrefe.

British Standards Institution (2026). BS 30480 Suicide and the Workplace. Available online at https://bit.ly/3IfGT4m (Accessed 18th December 2025).

British Standards Institution (2026). Suicide and the Workplace: A Practical First Steps Guide to Support. Available online at https://www.bsigroup.com/en-GB/insights-and-media/insights/brochures/suicide-and-the-workplace-a-practical-first-steps-guide/ (Accessed 18th December 2025).

BS 30480 Suicide and the workplace – Intervention, prevention and support for people affected by suicide: https://bit.ly/3IfGT4m

Suicide and the Workplace: A practical first steps guide https://www.bsigroup.com/en-GB/insights-and-media/insights/brochures/suicide-and-the-workplace-a-practical-first-steps-guide/

Davidson, J.E. and Richardson, M. (2023). *Workplace Wellness: From Resiliency to Suicide Prevention and Grief Management: A Practical Guide to Supporting Healthcare Professionals*. London: Springer.

Royal College of Psychiatrists (2022) Supporting mental health staff following the death of a patient by suicide – A prevention and postvention framework. Available online at: https://www.rcpsych.ac.uk/docs/default-source/improving-care/better-mh-policy/college-reports/college-report-cr234-staff-support-following-patient-suicide.pdf.

Samaritans – NHS Employee Suicide – A postvention toolkit to help manage the impact and provide support. Available online at: https://www.nhsconfed.org/system/files/2023-03/NHS-employee-suicide-postvention-toolkit.pdf.

University of Surrey, University of Birmingham and Keel University (ND) Postvention guidance – Supporting NHS staff after the death by suicide of a colleague. Available online at: https://www.surrey.ac.uk/sites/default/files/2024-09/postvention-guidance.pdf.

References

Abbate, L., Chopra, J., Poole, H. and Saini, P. (2024). Evaluating postvention services and the acceptability of models of postvention: A systematic review. *OMEGA-Journal of Death and Dying*. 90(2): 865–905.

Adshead, C., Runacres, J. and Kevern, P. (2025). Exploring the subjective experiences of peer-led social support groups for individuals bereaved by suicide. *Illness, Crisis & Loss*. 33(1): 44–61.

Ali, U. and Rehna, T. (2023). Grief reactions and suicide bereavement in the context of stigma among parents: An interpretative phenomenological analysis. *Annales Médico-Psychologiques*. 181(7): 598–603.

Ayala Romera, E.V., Sánchez Santos, R.M., Fenzi, G., García Méndez, J.A. and Díaz Agea, J.L. (2024). Emergency first responders' misconceptions about suicide: A descriptive study. *Nursing Reports*. 14(2): 777–787.

Bahamón, M.J., Javela, J.J., Ortega Bechara, A., Cabezas-Corcione, A. and Cudris-Torres, L. (2024). Attitudinal beliefs about suicidal behavior and attitudes towards suicide attempts in Colombian healthcare professionals. *Healthcare*. 12(21): 2169.

Bélanger, S.M., Hauge, L.J., Reneflot, A., Øien-Ødegaard, C., Christiansen, S.G., Magnus, P. and Stene-Larsen, K. (2024). General practitioner consultations for mental health reasons prior to and following bereavement by suicide. *Social Psychiatry and Psychiatric Epidemiology*. 59: 1533–1541.

Bell, J., Cunnah, K. and Earle, F. (2024). Understanding impact and factors that improve postvention service delivery: Findings from a study of a community-based suicide bereavement support service in England. *Mortality*. 30(4): 872–886.

Bride, B.E., Sprang, G., Hendricks, A., Walsh, C.R., Mathieu, F., Hangartner, K., Ross, L.A., Fisher, P. and Miller, B.C. (2024). Principles for secondary traumatic stress-responsive practice: An expert consensus approach. *Psychological Trauma: Theory, Research, Practice, and Policy*. 16(8): 1301–1308.

Calvo, S., Carrasco, J.P., Conde-Pumpido, C., Esteve, J. and Aguilar, E.J. (2024). Does suicide contagion (Werther effect) take place in response to social media? A systematic review. *Spanish Journal of Psychiatry and Mental Health*. S2950-2853(24): 1–11.

Causer, H., Muse, K., Smith, J. and Bradley, E. (2019). What is the experience of practitioners in health, education or social care roles following a death by suicide? A qualitative research synthesis. *International Journal of Environmental Research and Public Health*. 16(18): 3293.

Causer, H., Spiers, J., Chew-Graham, C.A., Efstathiou, N., Gopfert, A., Grayling, K., Maben, J., van Hove, M. and Riley, R. (2025). Filling in the gaps: A grounded theory of the experiences and needs of healthcare staff following a colleague death by suicide in the UK. *Death Studies.* 49(4): 448–459.

Causer, H., Spiers, J., Efstathiou, N., Aston, S., Chew-Graham, C.A., Gopfert, A., Grayling, K., Maben, J., Van Hove, M. and Riley, R. (2022). The impact of colleague suicide and the current state of postvention guidance for affected co-workers: A critical integrative review. *International Journal of Environmental Research and Public Health.* 19(18): 11565.

Čepulienė, A.A. and Skruibis, P. (2022). The role of spirituality during suicide bereavement: A qualitative study. *International Journal of Environmental Research and Public Health.* 19(14): 8740.

Cerel, J., Brown, M.M., Maple, M., Singleton, M., Van de Venne, J., Moore, M. and Flaherty, C. (2019). How many people are exposed to suicide? not six. *Suicide and Life-Threatening Behavior.* 49(2): 529–534.

Creegan, M., O'Connell, M., Griffin, E. and O'Connell, S. (2025). Exploring posttraumatic growth in individuals bereaved by suicide: A secondary data analysis of a national survey. *Death Studies.* 49(8): 1023–1103.

Dalum, H.S., Hem, E., Ekeberg, Ø., Reneflot, A., Stene-Larsen, K. and Hauge, L.J. (2024). Suicide rates among health-care professionals in Norway 1980–2021. *Journal of Affective Disorders.* 355: 399–405.

Erbuto, D., Berardelli, I., Sarubbi, S., Rogante, E., Sparagna, A., Nigrelli, G., Lester, D., Innamorati, M. and Pompili, M. (2021). Suicide-related knowledge and attitudes among a sample of mental health professionals. *International Journal of Environmental Research and Public Health.* 18(16): 8296.

Evans, A. and Abrahamson, K. (2020). The influence of stigma on suicide bereavement: A systematic review. *Journal of Psychosocial Nursing and Mental Health Services.* 58(4): 21–27.

Foggin, E., McDonnell, S., Cordingley, L., Kapur, N., Shaw, J. and Chew-Graham, C. (2016). GPs' experiences of dealing with parents bereaved by suicide: A qualitative study. *British Journal of General Practice.* 66(651): e737–e746.

Geleželytė, O., Gailienė, D., Latakienė, J., Mažulytė-Rašytinė, E., Skruibis, P., Dadašev, S. and Grigienė, D. (2020). Factors of seeking professional psychological help by the bereaved by suicide. *Frontiers in Psychology.* 11: 592.

Gibbons, R. (2023). Eight 'truths' about suicide. *BJPsych Bulletin.* 48(6): 350–354.

Gibbons, R., Brand, F., Carbonnier, A., Croft, A., Lascelles, K., Wolfart, G. and Hawton, K. (2019). Effects of patient suicide on psychiatrists: Survey of experiences and support required. *BJPsych Bulletin.* 43(5): 236–241.

Gilo, T., Feigelman, W. and Levi-Belz, Y. (2022). Forgive but not forget: From self-forgiveness to posttraumatic growth among suicide-loss survivors. *Death Studies.* 46(8): 1870–1879.

Goulah-Pabst, D.M. (2023). Suicide loss survivors: Navigating social stigma and threats to social bonds. *OMEGA-Journal of Death and Dying.* 87(3): 769–792.

Grafiadeli, R., Glaesmer, H. and Wagner, B. (2022). Loss-related characteristics and symptoms of depression, prolonged grief, and posttraumatic stress following suicide bereavement. *International Journal of Environmental Research and Public Health.* 19(16): 1–10.

Gutin, N.J. (2019a). Losing a patient to suicide: Navigating the aftermath. *Current Psychiatry*. 18(11): 17–24.

Gutin, N.J. (2019b). Losing a patient to suicide: What we know. *Current Psychiatry*. 18(10): 15–25.

Hansel, T.C. and Saltzman, L.Y. (2024). Secondary traumatic stress and burnout: The role of mental health, work experience, loneliness and other trauma in compassion fatigue in the healthcare workforces. *Traumatology*. 30(4): 615–618.

Hawton, K., Hill, N.T.M., Gould, M., John, A., Lascelles, K. and Robinson, J. (2020). Clustering of suicides in children and adolescents. *The Lancet Child & Adolescent Health*. 4(1): 58.

Hill, N.T., Robinson, J., Pirkis, J., Andriessen, K., Krysinska, K., Payne, A., Boland, A., Clarke, A., Milner, A. and Witt, K. (2020). Association of suicidal behavior with exposure to suicide and suicide attempt: A systematic review and multilevel meta-analysis. *PLoS Medicine*. 17(3): e1003074.

Huang, X., Ribeiro, J.D., Musacchio, K.M. and Franklin, J.C. (2017). Demographics as predictors of suicidal thoughts and behaviors: A meta-analysis. *PloS One*. 12(7): e0180793.

Ilic, M. and Ilic, I. (2022). Worldwide suicide mortality trends (2000–2019): A joinpoint regression analysis. *World Journal of Psychiatry*. 12(8): 1044.

Jones, P., Quayle, K.E., Kamboj, S.K., Di Simplicio, M. and Pitman, A. (2024). Understanding the influence of suicide bereavement on the cognitive availability of suicide: Qualitative interview study of UK adults. *Suicide and Life-Threatening Behavior*. 55(1): 1–12.

Jordan, J.R. (2017). Postvention is prevention - The case for suicide postvention. *Death Studies*. 41(10): 614–621.

Jordan, J.R. (2020). Lessons learned: Forty years of clinical work with suicide loss survivors. *Frontiers in Psychology*. 11: 766.

Kaspersen, S.L., Kalseth, J., Stene-Larsen, K. and Reneflot, A. (2022). Use of health services and support resources by immediate family members bereaved by suicide: A scoping review. *International Journal of Environmental Research and Public Health*. 19(16): 10016.

Kirchner, S. and Niederkrotenthaler, T. (2024). Experiences of suicide survivors of sharing their stories about suicidality and overcoming a crisis in media and public talks: A qualitative study. *BMC Public Health*. 24(1): 142.

Lenferink, L.I.M., Eisma, M.C., Smid, G.E., de Keijser, J. and Boelen, P.A. (2022). Valid measurement of DSM-5 persistent complex bereavement disorder and DSM-5-TR and ICD-11 prolonged grief disorder: The traumatic grief inventory-self report plus (TGI-SR+). *Comprehensive Psychiatry*. 112: 152281.

Lenferink, L.I.M., Van Den Munckhof, M.J.A., De Keijser, J. and Boelen, P.A. (2021). DSM-5-TR prolonged grief disorder and DSM-5 posttraumatic stress disorder are related, yet distinct: Confirmatory factor analyses in traumatically bereaved people. *European Journal of Psychotraumatology*. 12(1): 10.

Lestienne, L., Leaune, E., Haesebaert, J., Poulet, E. and Andriessen, K. (2021). An integrative systematic review of online resources and interventions for people bereaved by suicide. *Preventive Medicine*. 152: 106583.

Levi-Belz, Y. and Ben-Yaish, T. (2022). Prolonged grief symptoms among suicide-loss survivors: The contribution of intrapersonal and interpersonal characteristics. *International Journal of Environmental Research and Public Health*. 19(17): 10545.

Levi-Belz, Y. and Birnbaum, S. (2022). Depression and suicide ideation among suicide-loss survivors: A six-year longitudinal study. *International Journal of Environmental Research and Public Health*. 19(24): 16561.

Levi-Belz, Y., Krysinska, K. and Andriessen, K. (2021). "Turning personal tragedy into triumph": A systematic review and meta-analysis of studies on posttraumatic growth among suicide-loss survivors. *Psychological Trauma: Theory, Research, Practice, and Policy*. 13(3): 322.

Levi-Belz, Y. and Lev-Ari, L. (2019a). "Let's talk about it": The moderating role of self-disclosure on complicated grief over time among suicide survivors. *International Journal of Environmental Research and Public Health*. 16(19): 1–13.

Levi-Belz, Y. and Lev-Ari, L. (2019b). Attachment style and interpersonal facilitators as protective factors against complicated grief among suicide-loss survivors. *Crisis: The Journal of Crisis Intervention and Suicide Prevention*. 40(3): 186–195.

Marek, F. and Oexle, N. (2024). Supportive and non-supportive social experiences following suicide loss: A qualitative study. *BMC Public Health*. 24(1): 1190.

Morrissey, J., Higgins, A., Buus, N., Berring, L.L., Connolly, T. and Hybholt, L. (2024). The gift of peer understanding and suicide bereavement support groups: A qualitative study. *Death Studies*. 49(8): 1055–1066.

Murphy, P.T., Clogher, L., Van Laar, A., O'Regan, R., McManus, S., McIntyre, A., O'Connell, A., Geraghty, M., Henry, G. and Hallahan, B. (2019). The impact of service user's suicide on mental health professionals. *Irish Journal of Psychological Medicine*. 39(1): 74–84.

Nelson, P.A., Cordingley, L., Kapur, N., Chew-Graham, C., Shaw, J., Smith, S., Mcgale, B. and Mcdonnell, S. (2020). 'We're the first port of call' – perspectives of ambulance staff on responding to deaths by suicide: A qualitative study. *Frontiers in Psychology*. 11: 722.

Nic an Fhailí, M., Flynn, N. and Dowling, S. (2016). Experiences of suicide bereavement: A qualitative study exploring the role of the GP. *British Journal of General Practice*. 66(643): e92–e98.

Nicholas, A., Niederkrotenthaler, T., Reavley, N., Pirkis, J., Jorm, A. and Spittal, M.J. (2020). Belief in suicide prevention myths and its effect on helping: A nationally representative survey of Australian adults. *BMC Psychiatry*. 20: 1–12.

Niederkrotenthaler, T., Braun, M., Pirkis, J., Till, B., Stack, S., Sinyor, M., Tran, U.S., Voracek, M., Cheng, Q., Arendt, F., Scherr, S., Yip, P.S.F. and Spittal, M.J. (2020). Association between suicide reporting in the media and suicide: Systematic review and meta-analysis. *BMJ*. 368: 1–17.

O'Connell, S., Troya, M.I., Arensman, E. and Griffin, E. (2023). "That feeling of solidarity and not being alone is incredibly, incredibly healing": A qualitative study of participating in suicide bereavement peer support groups. *Death Studies*. 48(2): 1–11.

Ohayi, S.R. (2019). "Doctor, please don't say he died by suicide": Exploring the burden of suicide survivorship in a developing country. *Egyptian Journal of Forensic Sciences*. 9: 1–7.

Pearce, C., Wong, G., Kuhn, I. and Barclay, S. (2021). Supporting bereavement and complicated grief in primary care: A realist review. *BJGP Open*. 5(3): 1–11.

Peters, K., Cunningham, C., Murphy, G. and Jackson, D. (2016a). Helpful and unhelpful responses after suicide: Experiences of bereaved family members. *International Journal of Mental Health Nursing*. 25(5): 418–425.

Peters, K., Cunningham, C., Murphy, G. and Jackson, D. (2016b). 'People look down on you when you tell them how he died': Qualitative insights into stigma as experienced by suicide survivors. *International Journal of Mental Health Nursing*. 25(3): 251–257.

Pirkis, J., Bantjes, J., Gould, M., Niederkrotenthaler, T., Robinson, J., Sinyor, M., Ueda, M. and Hawton, K. (2024). Public health measures related to the transmissibility of suicide. *The Lancet Public Health*. 9(10): e807–e815.

Pitman, A., Osborn, D.P.J., Rantell, K. and King, M.B. (2016). Bereavement by suicide as a risk factor for suicide attempt: A cross-sectional national UK-wide study of 3432 young bereaved adults. *BMJ Open*. 6(1): 1–11.

Pitman, A., Osborn, D., King, M. and Erlangsen, A. (2014). Effects of suicide bereavement on mental health and suicide risk. *The Lancet Psychiatry*. 1(1): 86–94.

Prigerson, H.G., Singer, J. and Killikelly, C. (2024). Prolonged grief disorder: Addressing misconceptions with evidence. *The American Journal of Geriatric Psychiatry*. 32(5): 527–534.

Romero-Moreno, J.C., Cantero-García, M., Huertes-del Arco, A., Izquierdo-Sotorrío, E., Rueda-Extremera, M. and González-Moreno, J. (2024). Grief intervention in suicide loss survivors through cognitive-behavioral therapy: A systematic review. *Behavioral Sciences*. 14(9): 791.

Sandford, D.M., Kirtley, O.J., Thwaites, R. and O'Connor, R.C. (2021). The impact on mental health practitioners of the death of a patient by suicide: A systematic review. *Clinical Psychology & Psychotherapy*. 28(2): 261–294.

Sanford, R., Cerel, J., McGann, V. and Maple, M. (2016). Suicide loss survivors' experiences with therapy: Implications for clinical practice. *Community Mental Health Journal*. 52(5): 551–558.

Schlichthorst, M., Reifels, L., Spittal, M., Clapperton, A., Scurrah, K., Kolves, K., Platt, S., Pirkis, J. and Krysinska, K. (2022). Evaluating the effectiveness of components of national suicide prevention strategies: An interrupted time series analysis. *Crisis: The Journal of Crisis Intervention and Suicide Prevention*. 44(4): 318–328.

Spicer, L. (2024). Eye movement desensitisation and reprocessing (EMDR) therapy for prolonged grief: Theory, research, and practice. *Frontiers in Psychiatry*. 15: 1–7.

Spiers, J., Causer, H., Efstathiou, N., Chew-Graham, C.A., Gopfert, A., Grayling, K., Maben, J., van Hove, M. and Riley, R. (2024). Negotiating the postvention situation: A grounded theory of NHS staff experiences when supporting their coworkers following a colleague's suicide. *Death Studies*. 48(9): 937–947.

Spillane, A., Matvienko-Sikar, K., Larkin, C., Corcoran, P. and Arensman, E. (2019). How suicide-bereaved family members experience the inquest process: A qualitative study using thematic analysis. *International Journal of Qualitative Studies on Health and Well-Being.* 14(1): 1–12.

Suija, K., Rooväli, L., Aksen, M., Pisarev, H., Uusküla, A. and Kiivet, R. (2022). Coping with suicide loss: A qualitative study in primary healthcare. *Primary Healthcare Research & Development.* 23: e41.

Tamworth, M., Killaspy, H., Billings, J. and Gibbons, R. (2022). Psychiatrists' experience of a peer support group for reflecting on patient suicide and homicide: A qualitative study. *International Journal of Environmental Research and Public Health.* 19(21): 14507.

Till, B., Wild, T.A., Arendt, F., Scherr, S. and Niederkrotenthaler, T. (2018). Associations of tabloid newspaper use with endorsement of suicide myths, suicide-related knowledge, and stigmatizing attitudes toward suicidal individuals. *Crisis: The Journal of Crisis Intervention and Suicide Prevention.* 39(6): 428–437.

Treml, J., Nagl, M., Linde, K., Kündiger, C., Peterhänsel, C. and Kersting, A. (2021). Efficacy of an internet-based cognitive-behavioural grief therapy for people bereaved by suicide: A randomized controlled trial. *European Journal of Psychotraumatology.* 12(1): 1–14.

Wagner, B., Grafiadeli, R., Schäfer, T. and Hofmann, L. (2022). Efficacy of an online-group intervention after suicide bereavement: A randomized controlled trial. *Internet Interventions.* 28: 1–9.

Whitebrook, J. and Churchyard, J.S. (2025). 'You just wear a mask': An interpretative phenomenological analysis study to explore the impacts of bereavement by suicide among peer support group members. *Archives of Suicide Research.* 1–18

Whitebrook, J., Lafarge, C. and Churchyard, J. (2025). A suicide bereavement model: Based on a meta-ethnography of the experiences of adult suicide loss survivors. *Frontiers in Public Health.* 13: 1596961.

Witczak-Błoszyk, K., Krysińska, K., Andriessen, K., Stańdo, J. and Czabański, A. (2022). Work-related suicide exposure, occupational burnout, and coping in emergency medical services personnel in Poland. *International Journal of Environmental Research and Public Health.* 19(3): 1156.

8 Conclusion

Sarah Housden

This concluding chapter aims to bring together the ideas and tools explored across the book by summarising the ground covered through a brief guide to best practice for working with people affected by self-harm, or by thoughts of, or bereavement related to, suicide.

1. Where self-harm or suicidal thoughts are suspected, it is important to have that conversation, asking the person about what is going through their mind, and establishing how developed their plans are. Self-harm and suicidal thoughts are more commonly experienced than is sometimes realised and some people will find disclosure very challenging due to fear of stigma and concerns about what might happen if their thoughts and intentions are known. Forming a therapeutic relationship is important to gaining the trust of patients.

2. Remain interested in the stories of patients and service users, listening to their narratives with open and empathic responses. Asking "What is your story?" rather than "What is wrong with you?" is likely to establish a more trusting therapeutic relationship, leading to compassionate and collaborative interactions.

3. Although self-harm is less frequently disclosed by middle-aged and older people, a person's age does not exclude them from the risks associated with self-harm or suicide. It is important to remember that suicide amongst older adults (over 65s) is correlated with adverse childhood events (Sachs-Ericsson et al., 2016). There is no age or time limit on emotional distress, so we need to be open to hearing disclosures of self-harm or suicidal ideation from unexpected people a times.

DOI: 10.4324/9781003635611-9

4. When carrying out a risk assessment, be sure to describe the nature of risks in terms of the person's situation and what they are experiencing. When drawing up a safety plan, make sure this is a collaborative process, so that the plan has content that is meaningful to the individual. Acknowledge to the patient that while self-soothing, grounding, and distraction techniques will not solve the underlying problems, they will help them to move beyond the point of extreme emotional distress in this moment.

5. When describing a patient to colleagues or writing in notes, we need to say what we have seen, rather than our interpretation of it. A person who bangs their clenched hands on their own lap, and then on a table (see Alice in Chapter 3), could be dismissed as "aggressive", or alternatively, we can spend time seeking to understand their experience and what is frustrating them. Remember that how we label people tends to stay with them, even if they change.

6. As a healthcare worker, there is a likelihood that you and your colleagues may at some time be personally or vicariously affected by self-harm or suicide. Take time to understand people who have been bereaved by suicide, and to signpost them towards services that will have a specific understanding of their needs and experiences.

7. Be mindful of your non-verbal communication and especially of appearing to be hurried, as this can be an invalidating experience and can detract from the value of anything you say. At the same time, be particularly careful in your use of language, seeking to recognise and validate the distress a person is experiencing, regardless of whether we think an episode of self-harm is serious or not. To the individual, the build-up to all self-harm and the occurrence of all suicidal thoughts are likely to be incredibly distressing.

8. Remain engaged with wider social and systemic issues around equality and diversity. This includes, for example, understanding the effects of widespread discrimination against those of lower socioeconomic status, through disempowering systems and judgemental attitudes, which have been found to reduce access to specialist services and interventions.

9. Remain mindful of the history patients and service users bring to the relationship and how past experiences might impact the care we can provide. Be especially aware of the dangers associated with appearing to blame the person for the distress they are experiencing.

10. We can make a difference through our ability to develop meaningful relationships with our patients. Every clinical encounter has the potential to be therapeutic; each communication is a chance to move closer to recovery and healing. Being understanding and compassionate can save lives. This is a message of hope for all healthcare practitioners. Listen to service users and patients, asking sensitive questions that help them find the words to express what they are experiencing.

The Tools in Your Toolkit

As this book draws to a close, it is worth reflecting upon the tools and techniques now available to you, along with the understanding of self-harm and suicide. Your next step will be to find ways to begin implementing new understandings and skills into your everyday healthcare practice and interactions with patients.

Among other approaches, you should now have a clear understanding of the need to listen to people's experiences, and to support self-soothing, grounding, and paced breathing techniques, as well as having ideas for assessing risk and developing safety plans.

This book has also provided you with an understanding of therapeutic approaches which, while you are unlikely to implement with patients yourself, you may hear about or signpost them towards. These include Dialectical Behaviour Therapy, Cognitive Behavioural Therapy, Acceptance and Commitment Therapy, and Schema Therapy, alongside specialist self-help groups, support groups, and phone lines within the voluntary and charitable sector.

The overarching messages of this book include the need for compassion and understanding in our interactions with patients and service users, combined with a determination to use skills to help people hold onto hope in the most difficult circumstances. As non-specialist practitioners, working with people experiencing mental distress, you have an essential role to play in helping people to keep themselves safe, and in giving them the message that their lives are worth living. Equipped as you are with a range of tools to select from and share with patients and service users, we hope that your ability to help others will have increased through reading this book.

It is likely to be helpful going forward to spend time reflecting on what you have learned from this book, what actions you want to take forward for yourself from that learning, and what you may want to share with and pass on to others, remembering that understanding self-harm and suicide is important for us all: there is no "them" and "us" in healthcare.

Reference

Sachs-Ericsson, N.J., Rushing, N.C., Stanley, I.H. and Sheffler, J. (2016). In my end is my beginning: Developmental trajectories of adverse childhood experiences to late-life suicide. *Aging & Mental Health*. 20(2): 139–165.

Index

Note: **Bold** page numbers refer to tables.

Hewitt, J. 75
high-risk situation: managing
    professional anxiety in 116–119
hope: in crisis 109–125; inspiring 119;
    supporting suicidal people 109–125
hospital admissions and self-harm 10–11
"How" skill 36
hypothalamic-pituitary-adrenal (HPA)
    50–52, **51**

intense exercise 37
International Classification of Diseases
    11th Revision (ICD-11) 135

John, L. 15

Kiekens, G. 17
Klonsky, E.D. 73
Knapp, S. 93, 96
Kurtz, M. 29

language/terminology: healthcare
    practitioners 62–63; and self-harm 2–3
Lazarus, R. 33–34
Lifeline Australia 139
Linehan, M. 29, 31, 74, 82
listening: importance of 63; skills 64
longer-term approaches 140

Marshall, J.J. 98
Marzano, L. 95
Mental Capacity Act (MCA) 112–114, 124
Mental Health Act (MHA) 58–59, 112,
    113, 124; and capacity **113**
mental health crisis: after 121; goal
    planning 120–121; safety planning
    119–120
mindfulness practices 60
misunderstanding 62
myths relating to suicide loss 135

Nathan, R. 57
National Institute for Health and Care
    Excellence (NICE) 72, 77, 79, 83, 99

non-suicidal self-harm 3, 71–84; *see
    also* self-harm
non-suicidal self-injury (NSSI) 8, 17, 72
non-verbal communication 150
normalised harm 17

O'Connor, R.C. 76
Office for Health Improvement and
    Disparities 110
Office for National Statistics 110
O'Keeffe, S. 78
"opposite action" 39–40

paced breathing 37–38
Papageno effect 132
paramedics 133
parasympathetic nervous system (PNS) 51
passive suicidal thoughts 93–94
past experiences 30–33
past negative experiences: and self-
    harm 13; and suicidal thoughts 13
Pearlin, L.I. 53
peer support groups 138
post-traumatic growth (PTG) 135–136
post-traumatic stress disorder (PTSD)
    132, 139, 140
prevalence–presentation gap 19
primary care presentations 11–12
Process Model of Emotion Regulation 31
professional anxiety 124; factors
    increasing 117; managing in
    high-risk situation 116–119;
    reducing 117–118, 122
professional/practitioner response to self
    harm 1–2, 10–12, 18, 35–41, 80,
    93, 99, 111–112, 114, 118
professional support 60
progressive muscle relaxation 38
prolonged grief disorder (PGD) 132,
    135–136
Psychiatric Liaison Accreditation Network
    (PLAN) Model of care 118, 123
psychological understandings of stress
    53–55

For Product Safety Concerns and Information please contact our EU
representative GPSR@taylorandfrancis.com
Taylor & Francis Verlag GmbH, Kaufingerstraße 24, 80331 München, Germany